Food Allergies

Traditional Chinese Medicine, Western Science, and the Search for a Cure

Henry Ehrlich

Third Avenue Books

Cover by Christopher Lione

ISBN: 978-0-9843832-2-1

This book is printed on acid-free paper.

Printed in the United States of America

To Ella Jean

Contents

Acknowledgements

First, I must thank Dr. Xiu-Min Li of Mount Sinai School of Medicine for entrusting me with the privilege of telling the story of her work. I can't say enough about her and my esteem for her, but in the pages that follow, you will get the picture. I would also like to thank my co-authors Dr. Larry Chiaramonte and Dr. Paul Ehrlich for making me their collaborator over a long time, and imparting to me their inquisitive and patient-centered approach to medicine.

Next, Linda J. Miller, PhD; Arnold I. Levinson, MD; Anne F. Russell BSN, RN, AE-C; Jessica Martin, PhD; Mark Cullen, MD; and Adolph Singer, MD for reading the manuscript at various stages and offering suggestions, particularly on the credibility of the science, and its presentation.

Thanks, also, to Hugh Sampson, MD, who heads the Jaffe Food Allergy Institute at Mount Sinai, and his colleagues at Sinai Scott Sicherer, MD; Julie Wang, MD; Anna Nowak Wegzryn, MD; and Ying Song, MD, for talking to me about various aspects of the work. And to David Dunkin, MD and Jessica Reid-Adam, MD for discussing their very exciting research.

Dr. Renata Engler, has been especially helpful for her long-time appreciation in print and in person of Dr. Li's work, her incisive critique of the shortcomings of Western medicine in treating allergic disease, her framework for the possible incorporation of complementary and alternative medicine in American clinical practice, and for her spontaneous eloquence.

Thanks also to my old friend Tim Koranda for answering questions about Chinese culture.

Finally, I have enjoyed the support and advice of Susan Weissman, author of *Feeding Eden: the Trials and Triumphs of a Food Allergy Family*, the best memoir of negotiating the challenges of this epidemic I can imagine.

Dr. Li thanks the National Institutes of Health (NIH) for supporting her basic and clinic research, and FARE (Food Allergy Research and Education—formerly Food-Allergy Initiative for supporting her work into clinical trials. She is also very grateful to funds directly established at Mount Sinai School of Medicine including the Winston Wolkoff Fund for Integrative Medicine for Allergies and Wellness (Contributors: Stephanie Winston-Wolkoff and David Wolkoff, Barbara Winston, Ralph Lauren, Saks Inc.), Lisa Yu, the David L. Klein Jr. Foundation, Anna Sherbakova and Sergey Pichugov, Walter Alexander, Jonathan and Anne Garber, and Evan Fellman, Chris Burch Fund, Sean Parker Foundation, the Dugan family, and the Weissman family.

Foreword

John L. Lehr, CEO, Food Allergy Research & Education

My first awareness of the seriousness of food allergies occurred when I met my step-nephew Zach several years before I became the Chief Executive Officer of Food Allergy Research & Education (FARE), the nation's leading food allergy research, education and advocacy organization. Zach, who is now 14, is allergic to milk, egg, peanuts, tree nuts and shellfish. Soon after Zach became a part of my family, the daily challenges he had managing food allergies became apparent, as was the ever-present fear of anaphylaxis.

Since becoming CEO of FARE, I have met thousands of families struggling with the same issues and, tragically, a number of families who have lost their children to this insidious disease. Today, up to 15 million Americans are living with food allergies themselves and millions more when you include the accommodations made by their families and friends. While individuals take a number of precautions to successfully manage the disease, avoiding food allergens remains the only sure way to remain safe. Life-threatening reactions from accidental exposures are a reality, and the fact that a food allergy reaction sends someone to the emergency room every three minutes is a constant reminder of the need for a cure.

As the largest private funder of food allergy research in the world, FARE is committed to investing in science that will save lives. While food allergy research is still in the early stages, it is critical to explore innovative therapies and attract scientists from many fields and disciplines. Dr. Xiu-Min Li, a world-renowned scientist at Mount Sinai Medical Center, exemplifies those scientists.

In Henry Ehrlich's book *Food Allergies: Traditional Chinese Medicine, Western Science, and the Search for a Cure*, we follow Dr. Li's unique career as she investigates a potentially life-changing therapy for food allergies. The book reads like a medical thriller, as Dr. Li and her team explore an herbal formula developed from traditional Chinese medicine (TCM), and test this formula against the rigors of Western science. What ultimately follows is a deeper understanding of the complexities of human immunology, the interplay between TCM and Western medicine, and the dedication of the scientists who are working to solve this growing global health crisis. Although the author is a strict believer in laboratory and clinical research methods, and the importance of reporting research results in peer review journals, the patient stories Ehrlich presents at the end of the book offer anecdotal-but-compelling evidence of the promise of TCM as a viable therapeutic approach. Also in the thriller spirit, Ehrlich's book leads to a variety of exciting surprise endings including broader application of TCM in other diseases, explorations of possible avenues to alter the intergenerational course of allergies, and prospects for a unique vision of integrative medicine.

Well-written and easy-to-follow, this book will serve as a great reference for those interested in food allergies, clinical research, and the different pathways that may lead to a cure.

Introduction

I first met Dr. Xiu-Min Li in 2010 when I visited her office at Mount Sinai Medical Center in New York on the recommendation of Dr. Paul Ehrlich, my cousin, coauthor and cofounder of a website devoted to pediatric allergies and asthma. Paul is not normally inclined toward alternative treatments. In fact, our project with Dr. Larry Chiaramonte, another pediatric allergist—the publication of *Asthma Allergies Children: A Parent's Guide* simultaneously with the launch of asthmaallergieschildren.com and related ventures—deals forthrightly with the guideline medicine they both practice, although we do have a section on alternatives, which mentions Chinese medicine. Paul said he had heard Dr. Li speak and, because she was working in one of the world's top allergy-research institutions, thought it was worth trying to get Dr. Li to contribute to our site.

As a lifelong reader of the *New York Times*, my first acquaintance with traditional Chinese medicine (TCM) came on July 26, 1971, when the eminent columnist James Reston wrote about his emergency appendectomy while covering Henry Kissinger's visit to China.[1] The diagnosis and surgery were accomplished by a combination of TCM and Western medicine; however, his considerable postoperative pain was relieved by acupuncture. Reading it again 41 years later, I was impressed by how vibrant TCM was both as an academic and a practical field back then. My own association with TCM was confined to the jars of dried vegetables on shelves in Chinatown stores. The idea of treating allergies with TCM sounded like rebuilding New York's infrastructure with plans for the Pyramids, the Parthenon, and St. Paul's Cathedral—not to mention any engineering marvels in China itself.

Dr. Li's office is on the 17th floor of the Annenberg Pavilion at 100th Street and Madison Avenue. The drab built-to-last stain-resistant hallways leading from the elevator could be part of a research complex anywhere, with windowless laboratories on one side and offices on the other. Signs

1

point the way to biohazard showers. When I entered her office, however, I saw a panorama of Upper Manhattan sloping toward the East River, the water itself, and the Borough of Queens that reminded me of my old office at a bank farther downtown, where the views provided relief from my routine work of writing speeches for senior executives. Until then, it had never quite occurred to me that cutting-edge medical research could be conducted as well as finance in this setting.

Xiu-Min herself welcomed me warmly in her highly accented English, and we made a bit of small talk before I explained my mission, gave her a copy of our book, and asked her to talk about her work, which I had read about in a few newspaper articles.

She started by explaining that she not only did research but also ran an offsite clinic, treating mostly non-Chinese patients for allergic diseases—many with atopic dermatitis (eczema)—whom traditional allergists couldn't help. Her dream is that Western practitioners will be able to incorporate some of what she does into their work without necessarily learning the secrets of TCM—so-called integrative medicine.

It didn't take long for Dr. Li to convince me that she was on to something. One set of photographs in her computer made an instant impression. From left to right were four views of a little girl's feet. On the left, they were livid with eczema, which, I know from the occasional angry state of my own skin, can itch to the point of obsession. Kids and some grownups will scratch until their skin bleeds and gets infected. Paul has told me that when he was a resident at Bellevue, it was not uncommon for children to be hospitalized and their hands tied down to keep their fingers away from their sore skin.

Dr. Li's photographs showed steady improvement. By the third picture, the feet were largely clear, and in the fourth, not only was the skin immaculate, but the nails were polished. As the father of a daughter, I know about the role nail polish can play in a girl's life. The transformation from hated, painful objects to decorative ones was the best indication I could get that something significant had happened.

PART ONE

Background

The first two chapters define the nature of the problem and the context for Dr. Li's research. For many of us, food allergies seem to have come from nowhere, and are often dismissed by those who don't have them as the product of the medical imagination run amok, aided and abetted by indulgent parenting. However, it seems to me that food allergies are not something new, and that the potential for allergies is inherent. It can be elicited by certain interactions between our bodies and the environment, sometimes over generations, and sometimes much faster. The past few decades have seen the steady escalation of provocation to allergies of various kinds, culminating for now with food. Moreover, the medical response has been inadequate to the challenge, emphasizing avoidance, control of symptoms, and the suppression of the immune response. These shortcomings are particularly glaring when the patients are very young children consuming antigens that the rest of us eat with impunity. Times like these cry out for new directions.

1

An Epidemic of Progress

A child's eczema is usually the initial indication of the medical history that may lie ahead. It is the first step on what allergists call the "atopic [allergic] march" to be followed possibly by environmental allergies, asthma, and food allergies. These conditions seem to be escalating in number and severity with each new birth cohort, from baby boomers to generations X and Y, also known as millennials. The apparent explosion of life-threatening food allergies has focused attention on the problem, much of it quite unsympathetic.

Allergies are aggravating to both those who suffer from them and those who resent having to accommodate these patients.

Allergies are an epidemic (lots of people have them) but not a plague, in that they are not communicable and the fatality rates are relatively low. Asthma kills between 3 and 4 thousand Americans every year, and food allergies about 150,[2] many of whom also have asthma.

However, even nonlethal allergies disrupt the lives of children badly enough to make them overtired and inattentive in school, although the children are not usually sick enough to be kept at home. Allergic children are often demoralized to the point that their quality of life is significantly reduced, with long-term effect on learning and participation in normal activities. Similarly, the effect of allergic disease on adults results in reduced productivity and may damage employment prospects. Asthma costs the US economy an estimated $56 billion per year in medical outlays and lost productivity at school and work.[3] Allergic rhinitis, which most people call hay fever (although it has nothing to do with either hay or fever), affects between 10% and 30% of the population worldwide,[4] costing millions of days of school and work. Among asthmatic children in the United States, the prevalence of allergic rhinitis is 61%.[5]

Like other chronic diseases, allergies are stressful for families. Overseeing the patient's health often requires drastic alteration in diet and behavior. Siblings feel slighted, and so do spouses (almost invariably husbands, because mothers assume the responsibility for dealing with the allergies). Managing a food-allergic child costs American families an average of $4000 annually, only 20% of it in medical expenses; the bulk of the nonmedical expenses come in the form of the sacrifices that parents make at work in order to look after their children, according to a 2012 survey.[6]

Allergic reactions are prompted not by bacteria or viruses but by things that present most of us with no ill effects. Asked to accommodate a seriously allergic child, the nonallergic are often highly intolerant and dismissive. As I write this in the days leading up to Christmas, I have been reading about grandparents, aunts, and uncles of food-allergic children who would rather exclude families from holiday feasts than make considerations in their menus.

The explosive growth of food allergies leads many people to regard them as something new under the sun. The refrain from many of my contemporaries is "I don't remember anyone who was allergic to peanuts when I was a kid." Come to think of it, I don't either, but as the author Mark Jackson puts it in his invaluable book, *Allergy: The History of a Modern Malady*,[7] in ancient accounts of reactions to wasp and bee stings, the commonest types of "idiosyncratic reaction" were to foods. He cites the *Hippocratic Corpus*, written four hundred years BCE, which describes a "constituent of the body which is hostile to cheese, and is roused and stirred to action under its influence." Four centuries later, Lucretius wrote, "what is food to one, is to others biting poison." These observers ascribed the reactions to something in the people who reacted, not to the quality of the food. Clearly, the allergic mechanism was always there; it didn't just appear suddenly in 1990.

Allergies are "un-American." All the things that are blamed for the epidemic seem to emanate from our way of life. Greenhouse gases accumulating as fossil fuels are burned are making pollen seasons longer. Asthma gets much worse when the air is full of commerce—diesel particulates, car exhaust, and power-plant emissions. Better standards of sanitation protect us from bacterial infection, but when overdone, they may deprive our immune systems of the challenges they need to keep them in balance; otherwise-useful antibodies then prey on normally harmless proteins. Prolific use of antibiotics kills good bacteria as well as bad ones. Add to this the prevalence of sweet things in children's diets, which may further damage the digestive system, rendering it unable to break down complex proteins that then circulate in the blood as allergens. This indictment of modern living is known broadly as the "hygiene hypothesis."

Food allergens are overwhelmingly found in staples of American diets, especially kids' diets. The big eight allergens are peanuts, tree nuts, milk, eggs, fish, wheat, soy, and shellfish, some of which are frequently hidden in other foods. Peanuts are a special indignity. The anthem of baseball, our national pastime, cries, "Buy me some peanuts and Cracker Jack." Because Cracker Jack has peanuts in it, both of these are a problem to about 1.5% of our children. Jimmy Carter, the only American president since the 19th century to derive any income from agriculture, was in the peanut business. Peanuts are a great source of cheap protein, and that same protein turns out to be hazardous to many children.

New research[8] seems to support the idea that something about the United States makes children more atopic. Immigrant children are less allergic than American children, and having foreign-born parents seems also to afford some protection. The longer these children live in the United States, however, the more allergic they seem to become.

Allergies are not solely an American problem, however. Where "progress" goes, allergies follow, which is something Dr. Susan Prescott observed in her book *The Allergy Epidemic*.[9] Dr. Prescott is from Australia, where the rate of asthma is even higher than it is in the United States and where the financial costs of allergies are double those of arthritis. She contends that the immune system has adjusted to the modern world by subtle changes in DNA that cause it to treat otherwise harmless proteins as lethal intruders: "As allergic reactions are directed to the external environment, it makes sense that the areas of the body affected are those that are in most immediate contact with the environment: the skin, the airways and the gut." Thus, the allergic march—eczema, nasal allergies, asthma, and food allergies; as countries industrialize, these diseases march forward together.

Basics of Allergy

I will explain some of the basics of allergy now because the concepts are crucial for understanding what happens throughout the remainder of the book.

The word "allergy" was coined by the Viennese doctor Clemens von Pirquet in 1906 from the Greek *allos*, which means "different" or "other," and *ergon*, connoting energy or reactivity.[10]

The ability to distinguish things that belong in your body from those that don't is the foundation of the immune system. The immune system is not one thing but really a group of interlocking subsystems whose beneficial functions sometimes turn around and bite us. There are two principal components, the first being the *innate* immune system, which fights invaders but doesn't "remember" them. That is, each time the innate immune system encounters an infectious microbe or virus, it will attack it the same way, even if the body has been exposed repeatedly.

The other part is the *adaptive* immune system. This is the part that we learned about in high school. A first exposure to a virus such as smallpox can be deadly, but if by some miracle we survive, such a virus won't present a problem because we will have created antibodies that will recognize the virus and mobilize defenses that will kill it before it kills us. Dr. Jerome Groopman describes "the elegant choreography of [the T cells]…coordinating scores of enzymes and releasing a repertoire of proteins that, in the body, amounts to a solid wall of immune defense."[11]

Allergic reactions are a function of the adaptive system.

At the time of a *primary exposure* to an allergen, the immune system reacts in one of three ways, two of which are positive or harmless and the third of which is allergic. There are two kinds of helper T cells that come into play. These are Th1 (T-helper 1), which are associated with tolerance to allergens, and Th2 cells (T-helper2), which are associated with allergies. They signal to B cells, another class of white blood cells or lymphocytes, to produce antibodies called *immunoglobulins*, via a set of proteins called *cytokines*. The B cells are individually programmed to recognize a single antibody for a single antigen. When they get signals from Th1 cells, they produce an antibody called immunoglobulin G, or IgG. On our website we call it IgG[ood]. Th2 cells regulate production of the antibody IgE, or IgE[vil]. Both IgE and IgG are allergen specific. That is, each antibody is programmed to respond to a single allergen.

These antibodies bind themselves to receptors on *effector* cells—mainly *mast cells* (discovered in 1878 by, as we call him in our family, "the other Dr. Paul Ehrlich"—no relation) and *basophils*. The mast cells lodge primarily in the tissues where they are likely to encounter outside agents—

the skin, sinuses, lungs, and digestive tract. The basophils circulate in the blood.

Think of all the classic signs of an immune response in, say, a pimple that sprouts overnight—the redness and swelling caused by the release of fluid from the blood vessels in the region, pain as increased swelling stimulates local pain fibers, and heat. The body is trying to isolate and combat an infection from a clogged pore.

Then picture this same process happening inside you. When IgE-equipped cells encounter their target allergen, the chain of events we associate with an allergy attack commences. The mast cells release a "soup" of substances called *mediators* to attack it, the best known of which is histamine. When all this happens in your sinuses, you sneeze and get congested. When it happens in your lungs, you wheeze. With food allergies left untreated for even a few minutes, the process unfolds unpredictably in different parts of the body. An innocuous protein precipitates a full-scale inflammatory response. It's like calling 9-1-1 when your teenager forgets his house key and tries to enter the house through a basement window in the middle of the night: Once the cops arrive, mistakes can be made.

Three responses to primary exposure occur.

First is *immunization*. That is, the immune system will recognize an allergen but will react by producing IgG, courtesy of Th1, overwhelmingly a benign, protective antibody response against viruses such as smallpox and polio or bacteria, specifically a so-called blocking antibody called IgG4, which attaches itself to your effector cells. If your effector cells are equipped with allergen-specific IgG4, they will not release their toxins in the event that they encounter this allergen. There are tests available that show the presence of allergen-specific IgG. These do not mean you have an allergy (although there are those who contend otherwise, mostly vendors of fringe tests and therapies); they merely signify that you have been exposed.

Second is *tolerance*. There will be no clinical symptoms because the body can simply coexist with the substance, a kind of physiological "don't ask, don't tell" policy. Sometimes there is an initial immune response that becomes less and less with repeated exposures.

Third is *sensitization*. This response results from overproduction of the antibody IgE and a lack of regulation of the inflammatory response. It should be noted that high serum IgE levels—i.e., antibodies circulating in the blood—are not indicative of an allergy. They become a problem only if, as described above, they are mounted on effector cells. Normally, IgE should be the least abundant antibody in the blood—0.05% of all immunoglobulins.[12] A highly allergic individual will have many times more IgE than a nonallergic person. All those idle hands and so few natural enemies! The IgE antibodies don't have enough to do and start to recognize otherwise harmless or beneficial proteins as the enemy. The allergenic proteins associated with most serious reactions—Ara h1, 2, and 3* are the hardest to digest. They can withstand the onslaught of acids and enzymes that break down other proteins, including the weaker allergens Ara h6 and 8, gain access to the rest of the body through the stomach and the intestines, and possibly spark devastating reactions.[13]

It turns out that Ara h1 protein in peanuts is found in other things, including parasitic worms and insect venom, which provoke the immune system. Why do certain proteins end up in such disparate organisms? These shared elements are called "common protein domains," which are "part of a given protein sequence and structure that can evolve, function, and exist independently of the rest of the protein chain."[14] These common protein domains can also be plucked from one organism and grafted into the DNA of another, the basis of genetic modification, which frightens many of us, especially those with food-allergic children. Common protein domains have been identified in a variety of parasites, in multiple animal species, including cats, dogs, and people, and in plant species.[15]

Why do these proteins survive evolution? Let's just say they are there for a reason, such as storing energy or protecting from predators. Nature doesn't like to reinvent the wheel, either. Somewhere along the evolutionary continuum, these building blocks of life stayed the same even as some microorganisms diverged into plants and animals.

Origins of an Epidemic

Why have allergies increased exponentially in the past few generations? A new science called *epigenetics* is key to understanding what has happened, referring to "heritable changes in gene expression that are not due to changes in the DNA sequence." Subtle alterations in gene expression—

---

*Short for *arachis hypogaea*, Greek for "peanut."

what genes do and when they do them—are likely influenced by changes in environmental exposures. Genes themselves comprise only 2% of the genome, but the rest of the genome—which has been called "junk DNA"—contributes to the development of any organism in ways that have only recently come into focus.[16]

Some researchers describe the *epigenome* as the "clothing" of the genome, in which certain "layers change significantly during development and can be modified throughout life, whereas other layers remain relatively permanent." These differences help explain why individuals with the same or similar DNA—identical or unidentical twins, for example—may have very different health outcomes. Two important mechanisms contribute to this process by essentially sticking chemical "tags" on the DNA or the proteins that surround it, called *histones*. Methyl groups can be added to the DNA (this is called DNA methylation), which generally switches the gene "off," or histones can be chemically modified by the addition of acetyl groups, which leads to greater expression of the DNA. Conversely, the removal of methyl groups from DNA (demethylation) and acetyl groups from histones (deacetylation) switches genes "on."[17]

Families may be programmed by their DNA not to be allergy prone, but changes in gene expression can undermine that protection. Versions of this happen at each intersection of the body and the environment, as Dr. Prescott pointed out, and the changes in one generation can be passed to succeeding generations. UCLA researchers John S. Torday and Virender K. Rehan have found what they call a "smoking gun" linking grandmothers' smoking to asthma in their grandchildren.[18]

People who itch and sneeze seem to have children who wheeze, who then seem to have children who hive, swell up, collapse from plunging blood pressure, and asphyxiate upon eating certain foods.

Allergy treatment has generally been directed at symptoms, not at root causes. We take antihistamines when we sneeze and inhaled albuterol when we wheeze and try to steer clear of our triggers—the specific allergens that make us sick. Sometimes we use medicines prophylactically, such as antihistamines starting before the pollen season and inhaled corticosteroids to keep asthmatic inflammation under control, reducing the chance of an attack. (The inability to cure most allergies has made the pharmaceutical industry the center of a battle that long predates current frustration at the lack of progress; for a detailed account, see Mark Jackson's book.)

The closest we have to a cure is *hyposensitization*, consisting of multi-year programs of *immunotherapy*—also called allergy shots—which have been used to treat allergies for more than a century. The shots begin with small doses of antigen/allergen—a fraction of a unit—which are gradually increased until they reach a maximum or a maintenance dose. As IgE production is continually activated by introduction of the antigen, the cells that regulate production of new IgE (Th2 cells) are widely thought to become overloaded, and the quantity of IgE circulating diminishes proportionately with the amount of IgG4, the blocking antibody. As immunotherapy continues, these benign antibodies compete with IgE for available receptor sites on new mast cells in a kind of game of musical chairs, although once the antibodies are "seated," they don't get up again. Over time, with turnover of effector cells, the benign IgG antibodies dominate and allergenicity subsides. Now, another mode of therapy called *sublingual immunotherapy*—frequently called SLIT—in which the allergens are placed under the tongue, is growing in popularity, the idea of which parents find attractive for their kids. However, European doctors are more accepting of it than Americans. There are, moreover, reasons to doubt its effectiveness. [19, 20]

Shots haven't succeeded with food allergies, however. People with the worst food allergies are so sensitive that administration of even minute quantities of the allergen can provoke a deadly systemic response. That is what makes food allergies such a daily horror for millions of families. The big-eight food allergens are not only practically ubiquitous in standard American diets in their recognizable forms but are commodity additives to thousands of processed foods. A nonallergic child who eats tuna fish every day for lunch may be vulnerable from long-term exposure to mercury, but a dairy-allergic child also has to watch out for the milk protein *casein* that is sometimes added as a preservative.

Currently, numerous trials are underway at several research centers, usually coordinated under the Consortium of Food Allergy Research [COFAR][21] because of the difficulty of finding enough patients to take part, for courses of oral immunotherapy [OIT] for food allergies, an idea with a hundred-year history, in which escalating doses are consumed. (The Jaffe Food Allergy Institute at Mount Sinai in New York, where Dr. Li works, is prominent in these trials.) It remains to be seen, however, if the OIT trials, which have been promising for some patients, will result in lasting clinical unresponsiveness, as is the case with environmental allergy shots, or will have to be supplemented perpetually by regular doses of the allergen (as with insect venom immunotherapy). Mothers I correspond with say that their children will have to take eight peanuts a day for the rest of their lives after "completing" their OIT. The stakes are high. When seasonal allergens return, they are annoying; when anaphylaxis returns, the consequences can be tragic.

As Dr. Li puts it, "OIT doesn't fundamentally alter the immune system. The Th2 cells that regulate production of IgE may be stimulated to produce it until they are worn out, but new ones are created all the time. Without new allergen exposure to exhaust their IgE output in early stages, they may regain their strength." This happens with other forms of immunotherapy, such as rush immunotherapy for penicillin. When penicillin-allergic patients need antibiotics, they can be desensitized rapidly, which works long enough to receive treatment, but afterward, they will still be allergic and would require the same regimen the next time they need penicillin. It's one thing to receive rush immunotherapy, which you only need temporarily for an isolated medical procedure,[22] and another to spend months and months doing OIT for foods.

The distinction between desensitization and cure is critical. OIT may effectively raise the threshold of reactivity to reduce the possibility of accidental exposure, but whether it will permanently end the need for vigilance that food-allergic kids and their parents practice every day remains to be seen. Until it is, they must read labels minutely, avoid most restaurants, and carry powerful medication everywhere they go, all the behaviors that make food allergies so burdensome.

Another problem is that because IgE is allergen specific, it's hard to treat a patient for more than one food allergy at a time because of the danger of a serious reaction—one allergen may be tolerated fine and the other a problem, and the doctor wouldn't know which was which. That's why most of the studies of OIT are for only one allergen at a time (except for those studies that also use an "anti-IgE" medicine call Xolair—aka omalizumab—which costs $1000 a month and up for use with asthma). If, instead of desensitizing to one allergen at a time, we can modulate IgE in general until it is reduced to a normal, healthy fraction of immunoglobulin output, we would be much closer to a cure for food allergies while simultaneously treating "IgE-mediated" eczema, asthma, and environmental allergies.

An additional factor may be that anti-IgE omalizumab reduces the density of the high-affinity receptors on mast cells and basophils and makes them less sensitive to allergens.[23]

Dr. Li's research concentrates on the modulation side of that divide. She says, "We want to turn bad boys into good boys." She told me at that initial meeting two years ago, "It's not too early to talk about a cure." That was a surprise to me, because from everything I had read, it was far too early. Moreover, the fact that she was basing her research on combinations of herbs hundreds or even thousands of years old was counter to my own intuitions and ethnocentric biases. My conception of this kind of medicine was shaped by this exchange between Carl Reiner and Mel Brooks playing his classic character the 2000-Year-Old Man:

> Reiner: What did you do to stay healthy?
>
> Brooks: We had herbs, certain grasses, certain barks of certain trees…which are not to be mentioned on this record.
>
> Reiner: Why not?
>
> Brooks: Because I don't want to throw the entire ethical drug industry into chaos!

Little did I know.

Dr. Li spent five years starting in the late 1970s, not long after the universities were reopened, getting an MD in a Chinese medical school in Zhengzhou, where she studied both Chinese and Western medicines, and then another three years studying integrative clinical pediatric immunology in Beijing. After a year at Stanford, she had three years of additional training in clinical immunology at Johns Hopkins Medical School, working with Dr. Hugh Sampson. Dr. Sampson has been a leading figure in the effort to comprehend and treat the food-allergy epidemic since the 1980s. At Johns Hopkins, he led the effort to isolate the allergenic proteins in peanuts from 30 down to seven, among other things, and research into the possibility of injectable immunotherapy. Dr. Sampson is currently chief of the Division of Allergy & Immunology in the Department of Pediatrics, director of the Jaffe Food Allergy Institute, and dean of Translational Biomedical Science at the Mount Sinai Medical Center. He is also past president of the American Academy of Allergy, Asthma, and Immunology (AAAAI). His eventual decision to support Dr. Li's ideas may prove to be a pivotal event in the direction of allergy research and treatment.

After I met Dr. Li, I tried to get into the spirit of things and spent a few months reading about TCM with its thousands of years of tradition, belief systems, and alternative anatomy. I was bored. I don't believe that people can channel *Qi* (pronounced *chee*) and knock me over from across the room. And a philosophy that seems to boil down to "everything in moderation"—well, life is too short. Mine is, anyway.

The medical part of TCM is something else, though. In TCM literature, the formulas are directed at specific body parts and exhaustively described symptoms. They are also evocatively and poetically named; for example, the essential text *Formulas and Strategies* lists Cool the Bones Powder, which "clears heat from deficiency and alleviates steaming bone disorder," as does Sweet Wormwood and Soft-Shelled Turtle Shell Decoction Version 1.[24] (I wonder what the people responsible for names like Avastin and Celebrex would do with these medicines.)

If we can connect the classical TCM formulas with pathology recognized by Western doctors, we may get a head start on finding cures. As Dr. Scott Sicherer, professor of pediatrics and chief of Pediatric Allergy and Immunology at Mount Sinai School of Medicine, told me, "In China, what we call traditional Chinese medicine is just medicine. Western medicine looks at individual molecules to treat specific conditions, but it may be that many molecules or ingredients can do better and can affect the larger immune system. By looking at them one at a time, we may be missing out."

Enter Dr. Li.

The Ancient Origins of a "Modern" Affliction

We associate allergies with the industrialized world, but although the incidence of allergic diseases has increased exponentially over the past few generations, these tendencies have been there all along. When the Yellow Emperor began collecting remedies from Chinese doctors three thousand years ago, they were already treating symptoms that sound like allergies, and these remedies are still in use today. You don't have to believe that Prometheus brought fire from the heavens to know that you can use it to boil water.

Dr. Li sits between the two traditions like a Rosetta Stone, providing the key to translating the ancient into the modern. Studying her work and speaking to her colleagues, it's hard for me to escape the impression that she is a pivotal figure in medicine. She embodies a saying given to me by a Chinese-speaking friend: *tianshi, dili, renhe* (heavenly timing, location advantage, and human harmony), or, as we put it, being in the right place at the right time. I believe that if it hadn't been for the unique attributes of this individual, the integration of Western medicine and TCM would never have gotten as far as it has in this country, and, because she is so active on various national and international committees devoted to complementary and alternatives medicine, maybe in the world.

Dr. Julie Wang, one of Xiu-Min's colleagues at Mount Sinai who serves with her on those committees, is second-generation Taiwanese American. She was born and raised in the United States and educated in an American medical school. She said her only acquaintance with TCM was when she was growing up. "When I was sick, my grandmother would give me some herbal tea and say, 'This will make you feel better.'" Without the opportunity to work with Xiu-Min, TCM would never have entered Dr. Wang's professional life. Few people in the world have ever had the chance to study both disciplines in parallel. As far as I know, no one other than Dr. Li has had the precise scientific background and interest to delve into the mysteries of the immune system in this way, and no one else has had the combination of family and life circumstances that prepared them to take advantage of the geopolitical opportunities that have opened up in the past several decades. *Tianshi, dili, renhe,* indeed.

Dr. Li is very modest. She claims not to be an expert on all the disciplines that go into her work: "I am not a chemist, but I know enough about chemistry to direct the experiments." She is also not a statistician, but she knew enough about her own ambitions in research to study statistics, one of the critical tools, in medical school.

When I was trying to make sense of Chinese medicine in books, I thus took her at her word that it wasn't necessary to study the *meridians,* one of the tenets of TCM physiology, or to know which diseases, medicines, and foods are considered hot and cold, or which ones rise from the spleen or descend from the liver. But it is not enough to know that these medicines work. As Dr. Li and one of her many coauthors have written, "It is insufficient to investigate the clinical efficacy of CAM (complementary and alternative medicine) without giving priority to elucidating the mechanistic actions of these therapies. In food-allergy research, as we struggle to define the roles of specific immune cells, portals for allergen sensitization, and the role of food allergy in setting the stage for more severe allergic diseases later in life, it is important to incorporate what we learn from CAM into this paradigm."[25]

There are no Chinese molecules and Western molecules. Says Dr. Sicherer: "The good news for science is that this is being done by pharmaceutical protocols. Just because something is natural and it works doesn't mean it can be safely used. Dr. Li's work starts with safety before effectiveness, even though she has this body of medicine from China to draw on, and studies animals before humans. She meets all regulatory and ethical requirements."

In effect, Dr. Li's work starts from proven treatment and works from the bottom up to show why it is safe and effective. She and coauthor Laverne Browne, PhD, described the rigor of proof this way: "Unlike synthetic drugs that begin with preclinical laboratory studies, botanical drug development from TCM has the advantage of long-term experience in human beings and generally an established safe profile. However, standardization of herbal formulas is challenging because the complex mixtures of herbs contain many constituents that have not been clearly defined. An essential requirement for clinical investigation of a botanical drug is an IND [investigational new drug] approval by the FDA (Title 21 Code of Federal Regulations 312.23 (a)). The most unique section in this IND is the Chemical, Manufacturing, and Control (CMC) Data [21 CFR 312.23(a) (7)] requirement, which differs from that required for synthetic drugs. Given the unique characteristics of herbal mixtures, the FDA frequently relies on a combination of tests when the active chemicals are not well defined. HPLC [high-performance liquid chromatography] fingerprints, assays of characteristic markers, and biological assays are accepted methods to ensure quality, potency, and consistency of botanical drugs."[26]

What is the alternative from Western medicine? I read about the full spectrum of allergic diseases all the time and have somehow managed to enlist leading scientists and practitioners in writing for our website. Insights into the mechanisms of allergy are exploding. There is a lot of good science, but somehow, articles with titles like "Anti–IL-5 Therapy Reduces Mast Cell and IL-9 Cell Numbers in Pediatric Patients with Eosinophilic Esophagitis [EoE]" don't point to anything like a broad-based "cure" in the foreseeable future. Even if a convenient way to synthesize anti-IL-5 agents and administer them to patients were found, it would be years before we knew whether it constituted an effective therapy for EoE, a potent and painful allergy of the digestive system, and at what cost. Synthetic antibodies to allergic effector cells are massively expensive.

The road from clinical insight to useful treatment is very slow. In 2012, I heard Dr. Arnold Levinson of the University of Pennsylvania challenge an audience of allergists to name a single real breakthrough in asthma treatment since the development of inhaled corticosteroids in 1944, which really only became economical with the discovery of the active ingredient *diosgenin* in wild Mexican yams in 1980.[27] No one raised a hand.

Standard allergy treatment is effective as far as it goes, but to a great extent, it just continues the stalemate treatment of the past hundred years, and for food allergy, it offers very little. With the rate of food allergies tripling over the past ten years, particularly peanut allergy, which is outgrown only 20% of the time, we face a crisis of accommodation in schools and restaurants, to name just two. Long term, institutions such as the military will be foreclosed to large numbers of otherwise qualified recruits, as Dr. Anna Nowak-Wegrzyn of Mount Sinai has written.[28]

Many parents are taking matters into their own hands by forking over large sums to allergists who offer desensitization through OIT even though it is regarded as experimental and not FDA approved. I am sympathetic to these parents because OIT, although not a cure, does seem to offer limited protection against accidental ingestion for some people.

If a willingness to pay out of pocket for OIT is one measure of how anxious families are for relief from the day-to-day battle, so is their openness to alternative medicine. Large numbers of families have sought alternatives, although the numbers reported vary from one study to another. The 2002 National Health Information Survey showed that 36% of adults used CAM—"62% if prayer was included."[29] A 2006 survey[30] of patients generally, not just for allergies, found that unproven or disproven diagnostic methods and (CAM) were used by approximately 20% of respondents, although they weren't impressed with the results. The survey also found that, given a choice, many would prefer herbal therapies to pharmaceutical drugs. By 2009, there were reports that 62% had used a CAM treatment and 26% had done so at the suggestion of a physician. Many of these responses undoubtedly included recommendations to use certain vitamins, which, like prayer, fall under the broad heading of CAM.[31]

Patients seeking a path between mainstream and alternative medicine are often hamstrung by doctors' unwillingness to explore these options, however. Patients with allergic diseases are more likely to seek alternative treatments than those with any condition other than lower back pain.[32] As Dr. Renata J. M. Engler has written:

It has been easier to ignore the whole area of CAM as "placebo" or "not effective" and many patients complain that it is difficult to find a health care provider willing to partner with alternative practitioners or to monitor them if they choose an herbal or other CAM therapeutic trial outside the Food and Drug Administration–approved pharmaceutical industry.[33]

This does provide an opening for TCM, particularly as health-care costs have grown exponentially. As Dr. Li and Julia Ann Wisniewski, MD, one of her many collaborators, have written, "we have an obligation to our patients to understand their reasoning and interest in complementary treatments and to help them to make educated decisions about the potential risks and benefits of each. For patients with severe disease and limited conventional therapeutic options, or for those who have suffered from unwanted side effects of conventional therapies, we should break the cultural and social barriers to accessing complementary therapies that have been proved to be safe and beneficial."[34]

Dr. Li's team turns ordinary mice into peanut-allergic mice by feeding them a combination of cholera toxin and crushed peanuts. Then they use herbal concoctions to reverse the process. They have completed their animal studies, and as you will read, are now in human trials.

This research is conducted in compliance with the standards set by the National Center for Complementary and Alternative Medicine (NCCAM) of the National Institute of Health (NIH). Although many critics contend that NCCAM began as cover for the supplement industry, successive legislation has made it a sponsor and watchdog for rigorous research such as Dr. Li's and may provide a pathway to market for effective treatment at a lower cost than standard pharmaceuticals. The record of NCCAM-supervised research has been more productive for what has been disproven than what has been proven. Dr. Craig Hopp, Program Officer, NCCAM, said in an email to me:

> NCCAM-funded research in the natural products field has yielded limited data, if any, regarding products with 'proven' efficacy. While we have seen some positive results regarding omega-3s, and hints of promise with other natural products in basic and pre-clinical research, to date, most of our large, randomized, placebo-controlled, clinical trials in this area,

such as the Ginkgo Evaluation in Memory Study (http://nccam.nih.gov/research/results/gems), have not demonstrated greater efficacy versus placebo for the products, populations, and conditions studied.

As a nonscientist, I have struggled to understand the story of this research. I have slogged through dozens of peer-reviewed articles. When I started paying attention to medical literature a few years ago, I mentioned to a friend who is a public health authority and a department head at a major medical school that I read the abstracts and the discussion and couldn't make much sense of everything in between. He said, "That's all any of us do." But for this project I did my best with the middle, too. There is a complex set of characters at work: not the scientists who did the work—this is not *The Double Helix*, which recounted the human drama behind the great discovery—but the many cells that comprise the immune system and the processes that regulate our health.

Although I deeply understand the impatience for a cure, I also have more respect and understanding for the rigors of the scientific method than ever before. Many mice have died, but human lives will be saved.

2

The Parasite-Food Allergy Connection

U nlike asthma and other allergic diseases, food allergy is not described in the TCM literature.[35] When Dr. Li did her training in the 1970s and 1980s, it wasn't part of her curriculum. Even today, food allergies, particularly peanut allergy, are less common in China than in "industrialized" countries. By one account, the raw numbers of peanut-allergic people in China are today estimated to be the same as in the United States, even though the population is four to five times as large. Roasting, the standard US cooking method, is thought to make peanuts more aller-genic than boiling, frying, or pickling, which are more common elsewhere, because it leaves the allergens intact, whereas the other cooking methods partially denature them.[36]

TCM practitioners have been treating related diseases—allergic rhinitis, eczema, and asthma—for millennia with no clear idea of what the underlying mechanisms were, however; the antibody IgE was only identi-fied in the late 1960s, by US researchers. When Xiu-Min came to New York from Johns Hopkins with Dr. Hugh Sampson to work at Mount Sinai, she established an outside clinic that would specialize in eczema. "People with bad eczema have a very low quality of life, and I thought that US med-icine, which only treats the skin itself, wasn't adequate. If it's really bad, doctors do give oral prednisone, but that has side effects for the immune system overall.

"I had treated lots of eczema at the Chinese–Japanese Friendship Hospi-tal in Beijing, where we treat it internally as well as topically, because there are different things that cause it. Even so, I was unprepared for the severity I saw. Dr. Sampson sent me two patients who were covered head to toe. There was no clear skin. It seemed to me that there were several different causes, so I had

20

to prioritize and treat them all. The first thing was to bathe patients with herbal extracts, then use skin creams that were adapted from salves for treating wounds and burns, and when the skin started to show improvement, different skin creams and herbal tea."

The clinic practice built by word of mouth, and as the patient rolls grew, more and more patients presented with multiple food allergies, asthma, and sky-high IgE.

Back in the laboratory at Mount Sinai, food-allergy research focused on immunotherapy. Dr. Li says, "Dr. Sampson and I had been working on different kinds of peanut vaccine using animal models. In one study, we collaborated with Dr. Wesley Burks to investigate if a plasmid DNA*-encoding Ara h2 gene therapy could prevent peanut anaphylaxis. Our idea was that if mouse host cells express Ara h2 gene and make Ara h2 protein, the immune cells may believe that Aha h2 is their own protein so that they would not react against it."

Instead of inducing any protection, however, "We actually made the mice more prone to anaphylaxis. Normally, negative data would not be published, but we submitted our findings to *Journal of Immunology*, and the manuscript was accepted without revision.[37] We continued to collaborate with Dr. Burks and made engineered Ara h2 gene construct and then Ara h1 and 3 by modifying the Ara h1, 2, and 3 gene sequences. Our hypothesis was that the modified proteins would not be recognized by the IgE on the mast cells so that they would not cause reactions. We did see protection, but only partially, and only if the modified proteins mixed with heat-killed *Listeria monocytogenes* or *E-coli* bacteria as adjuvants. These immunotherapeutic approaches cannot be given orally; they require subcutaneous or rectal administration. Before I had the idea to test Chinese herbs, we had tested at least 10 different types of immunotherapy."

The focus of her research changed when she sat with mothers of severely food-allergic children at a fundraising dinner. After Dr. Li described the excellent results she was getting with the herbal treatments for eczema, one of the mothers told Dr. Li about her daughter's food allergy and said she hoped Dr. Li could someday do the same with children like hers. After listening to this story and speeches by other mothers that

---

*Genetic structure on a cell that can replicate independently of the chromosomes.

21

were just as touching, Dr. Li says, "From that moment, I felt that as a physi-cian-scientist, I had obligation to find a cure for these families. None of our tested immunotherapy was satisfactory in mouse models, which didn't hold out much promise for eventual human treatment. This is one of the reasons that I started to look for the potential of Chinese herbal medicines."

Xiu-Min began studying the symptoms these mothers described, and something sounded familiar. She says, "I had memorized hundreds of for-mulas that used 500 different herbs. The connection with food allergies was blurry at first, but the symptoms began to sound like parasites."

She presented her ideas to Hugh Sampson, who told me, "At that point, I was interested in anything that might be used to treat food aller-gies." Unfamiliar with the Chinese tradition, he was skeptical but never-theless gave the go-ahead with the condition that he would be active in the research at every stage.

Dr. Renata Engler is forthright in her appreciation of Sampson's deci-sion. She says, "Given that there was nothing else new, Dr. Sampson's vision to pay attention to the long, anecdotal track record was precedent-breaking." As the work went on and started to show promise, Dr. Sampson worked with donors to direct more resources to it.

Intestinal parasites had played a key part in Dr. Li's early medical career. As a teenager, she had spent a couple of years in the mid-1970s in a farming village as a barefoot doctor, a job created in postrevolutionary China because medical care was so scarce, and the worms were a big part of her work. James Reston wrote in his 1971 article about his own experi-ence with Chinese medicine: "Dr. William Chen, a senior surgeon of the United States Public Health Service [said] that before the Communists took over this country in 1949, four million people died every year from infectious and parasitic diseases and that 84 per cent of the population in the rural areas were incapable of paying for private medical care even when it was available from the 12,000 scientifically trained doctors."

Parasites are nasty. When they establish themselves in the intestines, they irritate or even perforate the lining, leaving it vulnerable to penetra-tion by large undigested molecules.

Formulas and Strategies, mentioned earlier, describes what happens:

> [I]ntermittant periumbilical (around the navel) pain...change in the complexion (usually wan, pale, or

dark)…white spots in the malar (cheek) region, night-time grinding of teeth, indeterminate gnawing hunger, vomiting of clear fluids.…If the condition is treated improperly and persists long-term, the patient will become emaciated and listless, lose interest in eating, and develop poor vision and hearing, dry hair, and a large distended abdomen. Infestation by parasites is a common cause of childhood nutritional impairment.

The life cycle of roundworms is as follows: Eggs pass through the stomach to the upper intestine, where they hatch into larvae. These burrow through the intestines, enter the bloodstream or lymphatic system, and end up in the lungs, where they mature. Nine days after ingestion, the time it takes for the larvae to pass from the lungs, up the airways, and into the mouth, they may be swallowed again and their life cycle repeated. The process from swallowing the eggs to having mature worms in the small intestine can take between two and three months, causing plenty of damage.

Parasites are nature's extortionists. Dangerous though they are, they are not ordinarily fatal. As with loan sharks and blackmailers, it is not in their interests from an evolutionary point of view to kill their hosts, just feed off them. Patients who survive an initial exposure have a defense in the form of IgE antibodies attached to their mast cells and basophils, which are on guard against re-exposure, or, in the case of most parasites, regeneration.[38] Children are most at risk because their immune systems are too immature to get them through the initial exposure.

In contemplating the power of IgE as a weapon of food-allergy destruction, it helps to know how it works as nature intended it, as a defense against parasites, which can cause an increase in total serum IgE of 10 to 100 fold.[39]

A study by Harvard researchers compared a group of "wild-type" mice to a control group that had been bred to be IgE deficient. As the name "wild-type" implies, these are mice that are held close to natural, not laboratory hybrids. They were all infected with *trichinella spiralis*, which causes trichinosis, known to chefs everywhere as the reason we don't serve rare pork. It kills about 50 people a year in the United States, usually from undercooked wild game as well as pork.

The wild-type animals mounted a robust IgE response that peaked on day 14 after primary infection, and the scientists concluded that "the role of IgE in immunity to *T. spiralis* is not restricted to facilitating the expulsion of adult worms from the intestine but also includes killing of larval stages of the parasite."[40]

The authors of this study concluded that their work "provides support for the long-held but disputed notion that parasitic infections have provided the evolutionary pressure that has selected for the persistence of the IgE-Fc RI system." (Fc RI refers to the "high-affinity receptors" on effector cells to which IgE attaches while waiting for the antigens that will cause them to unleash the barrage of histamines and other mediators.)

In trying to visualize this mechanism in a food-allergic person, remember that intestinal worms are complex, multicelled animals, not a few isolated proteins. The immune response for such an intruder must be powerful and persistent. Now picture this same attack mobilized in response to a bite of a Reese's peanut butter cup.

TCM treatment for parasites augments natural defenses by paralyzing the worms and disrupting their reproductive cycle so they can be expelled before they can implant new larvae, while at the same time quelling destructive inflammation and relieving pain.

The chosen instrument of the initial effort was the nine-herb traditional formula *Wu Mei Wan* (WMW). According to Dr. Li, WMW was classically prescribed "for colic, vomiting, chronic diarrhea or dysentery, and collapse (also translated as syncope) caused by parasitic worms. WMW has also been recently reported to be effective for treating several other syndromes, such as drug-induced rash, neurogenic vomiting, asthma, chronic gastroenteritis, and colitis."[41]

To the basic formula, two more ingredients particularly effective at immobilizing worms were added: *Zhi Fu Zi* (pharmaceutical name *Radix Lateralis Aconiti Carmichaeli Praeparata*) and wild *Ling Zhi* (*Ganoderma lucidum*, also known as *reishi* mushroom). (More about *Zhi Fu Zi* in a later chapter.) *Ling Zhi* of the quality Dr. Li wanted to use is rare and required using personal connections in China to locate a reliable supply in a remote, pristine region.

The new formulation was designated FAHF-1—short for Food-Allergy Herbal Formula-1.

Dr. Li told me that *Ling Zhi* has a special place in the TCM formulary and that it is mentioned in one of China's most treasured folktales, about a white snake that is turned into a beautiful woman. I asked a friend—the same one who gave me the proverb mentioned in chapter 1—about this story. He remarked that his father-in-law had played in the orchestra when the opera was performed at the Beijing Opera. He gave me a web link to a coherent retelling of the story where I found clues to the properties of the magic herb pertinent to treating food allergies.

Having been transformed from a white snake into Lady White, the newly formed woman meets a young man. They fall in love and marry. An abbot from a local temple, however, is on to her. During an annual festival devoted to driving away snakes, he urges this woman to take part in the ritual by drinking ritual *realgar* wine. She resists because she knows that it will turn her back into a snake, but she eventually agrees to drink to please her husband, with bad results. She passes out and reverts to a snake, whereupon her husband "dies" of shock. When she resumes her beautiful human form, she wakens, and seeing that her husband is dead, she declares, "I will fly to Kunlun Mountain and steal a miracle mushroom from the gods. That and nothing else can bring him back to life."

This being a fairy tale, there is a battle with enchanted animals guarding the mushroom, and other supernatural obstacles, but she secures a sample and returns home, where she feeds her husband a drink made from it. He is revived.

Still, although he is ignorant of events that took place while he was "dead," the husband is shaken, and it is only after a period of struggle that he and Lady White eventually live happily ever after.

Like many folktales, this story reveals truths about the world and society in which its creators lived, and observations about cause and effect that could be called scientific. It shows the centrality of parasites in community and personal health, and the value that people attached to treating them.

The part that really got to me, however, was the fact that the couple's lives are changed by the experience, and not for the better. The husband becomes tentative and fearful. This brush with death suggests anaphylactic shock, when the blood pressure plunges and the airways become constricted and fill with mucus. In autopsies, this is virtually indistinguishable from fatal asthma.[42] The stamp of anaphylaxis on the lives of contemporary food-allergic families is indelible, particularly when the patient is a child.

As I have learned by communicating with many distraught mothers, once the threat of anaphylaxis enters the lives of families, the world changes. It becomes dark and ominous, and each casual ingestion of certain foods can be life threatening. The more I deal with food-allergic patients and particularly their mothers, the more I hear the echo of the tale of the white snake.

To a TCM practitioner also trained in Western science, as Dr. Li is, this is much more than a folktale about a folk cure. *Proving* the efficacy of classic formulas, *disproving* them (which is also part of science), and *improving* them is the focus of robust research in China. As Reston put it, "like everything else in China these days, it is on its way toward some different combination of the very old and the very new." I can't think of any more apt example of how very old and very new are being combined than in the promise that TCM holds for curing incurable diseases.

PART TWO

The Science

These chapters primarily recount a series of painstaking experiments, starting with the creation of an animal model for testing, as well as explanations of other facets of the modern scientific method. They are followed by discussions of several newer lines of research that aren't complete yet but that indicate exciting new directions the science may take.

Until I made my way through the published articles, I had little appreciation for the conventions of scientific publishing, which involves recapitulating the background to the current experiment using the same or similar words and citations. To an amateur researching a particular area, they do appear to cover the same ground over and over again, often in the same or similar words, and cite the same references before getting to anything new. It's as if the Twelve Days of Christmas became the six months of Christmas and you had to sing every verse just to get to the next one. However, as Linda Miller (a PhD immunologist, a postdoctoral fellow at the National Cancer Institute, founding editor of *Nature Immunology*, and, incidentally, another cousin) explained to me that papers are written this way to both provide formal structure to thinking and facilitate experimental replication. Recapping the history in similar words and citations may be repetitious, but it provides background, continuity, and context: "For replication, identical or similar experiments are initially performed to make sure your system is aligned with previously published work so that your new experiments proceed on a proven foundation."

Replicability is everything, one of the main principles of the scientific method, as my trusty Wikipedia reminds me. With all the scandals of the past several years about the quality of published research, I have begun to find this repetition reassuring, especially considering the pioneering nature of the work. Replicability lay at the heart of Dr. Sampson's determination to oversee the research with a skeptical eye. This was alien territory. It wasn't enough to show good data. He says, "I had the researchers repeat the experiments several times. The results were consistent; they utilized the appropriate science and hit all the standard immune markers."

Dr. Li's herbal formula is now the most advanced investigational drug in the history of the NCCAM. A great deal is riding on it, and the methods must be meticulous. The results of each study must not only satisfy the researchers but also their reviewers at the NIH.

Although I have done my best to clarify the literature, it is often tough sledding, full of obscure numbers and Greek letters. Sometimes it's hard to tell the interferons from the interleukins, and the T cells from the B cells, and so I thought it might be useful to have a preview of the chapters that follow.

3. Establishing a Suitable Animal Substitute for People in Research

Oviously, you can't try this on human beings, and you can't wait around for lab animals to evolve the full set of deadly immune-system vulnerabilities as people. Mice are well established for this kind of research, but the challenge remained of inducing allergies using forced feeding of peanut extract with the help of a reagent to speed up the process, then determining whether the physiological responses were close enough to human responses to continue to use them in later work. Each time a new experiment commenced, it began with the same strain of mice and identical procedures.

4. A First Test of Efficacy—FAHF-1

FAHF-1 was a "beta version" of the food-allergy herbal formula. The classical version of WMW that constitutes the basis for this treatment contains ingredients that raise some regulatory red flags for use in humans but were adequate for testing in mice. Even in this version, the experiment showed that the drug could be administered safely, that it mitigated allergic symptoms, including the most serious (anaphylaxis), and that the biochemistry associated with these changes could be studied. Most important, here was convincing evidence that a Th1-Th2 imbalance might be correctible, that an allergic immune system could be "cured."

5. Process of Elimination

This chapter covers the thinking behind the regulatory concerns about a couple of the ingredients in the classic formula. The substitutions and recalibrations may surprise you.

6. Proof

This chapter recounts two experiments that not only demonstrate the efficacy of FAHF-2 on all key measures but also, for the first time, show that the curative effects last well past the cessation of therapy.

7. Whole Greater Than the Sum of Its Parts

When you start with an ancient formula arrived at through centuries of trial and error, you have to wonder if modern science might reveal some shortcuts. Maybe fewer herbs might yield the same results, which would make the whole process of gathering the ingredients, refining, and packaging that much simpler and cheaper. To that end, each of the ingredients was tested individually. The medicinal properties were studied, and it was revealed that in fact, the whole package was more effective than any lesser combination.

8. How Long Does It Last?

This chapter explores what amounts to a philosophical divide in food-allergy treatment as well as a medical one—the desirability and efficacy of oral immunotherapy for food allergies to desensitize them and raise the threshold of accidental ingestion on the one hand compared to lasting correction of the immune system on the other. The Mount Sinai teams shows that "*In vivo* (in the live mice) and *in vitro* (in a laboratory culture) this was the first evidence that an herbal formula can produce complete, long-lasting protection against peanut-induced anaphylaxis."

9. Contemplating Human Trials

Research doesn't follow a straight line. Before they were done with the mice, the Sinai team began to plan for the day when they could safely begin to work with people. This entailed thinking about what form, liquid or pills, would work best, and then showing whether, apart from efficacy, FAHF-2 could be administered without harming human subjects.

10. Too Many Pills

Even a "miracle cure" is useless if patients can't stand to take the medicine. In transforming WMW from a centuries-old herbal treatment into a 21st century medicine, the researchers had to consider Western tastes and customs. As anyone who has been told to continue a course of antibiotics even after starting to feel better knows, medication fatigue is a real thing. Brewing tea from a combination of herbs in quantity and drinking every day would be a burden for American mothers and kids. Pills are better—but how many?

11. Documenting the Quest for a Cure

Researchers must document annually all investigational drugs regarding how far they have come, where they plan to go, and how they intend to get there. This chapter provides the snapshot of progress taken in October 2012 showing how human subjects have reacted and describing procedures for the next phase of trials.

3

Establishing a Suitable Animal Substitute for People in Research

In 1945, writer E. B. White published the classic children's novel *Stuart Little*, in which a New York woman gives birth to a very unusual child—a mouse with the intellect and feelings of a human being. White was prescient. Genomics research has revealed to us that mice and humans have considerable genetic overlap. According to a 2010 European Commission paper, "99% of human genes are conserved in mice." Although other animals—dogs, pigs and primates, particularly—have even more in common with people than mice do, this same paper pointed out, "Working with these large animals is extremely expensive and is fraught with ethical concerns"—not to mention the logistical nightmare of transporting large numbers of them to the 17th floor of the Annenberg Pavilion at Mount Sinai. The small size and short generation times of mice, ease of breeding and keeping, and decades of their use in research have given scientists detailed understanding of mouse biology and genetics.[43]

Despite long use of TCM compounds with human patients, the researchers at Mount Sinai had to demonstrate the safety and efficacy of those compounds in animals according to exacting protocols. Whether applying to the NIH or the Department of Defense (DoD), which sponsor most basic research, these are your tax dollars at work. Dr. Li says regulators don't want too much novelty. Writing grant proposals and gaining scarce funding is an orderly process, and the NIH shies away from research that involves too great a leap; likewise, peer-reviewed journals. The closer a project gets to market, the larger the share of support must be gathered from nongovernmental sources.

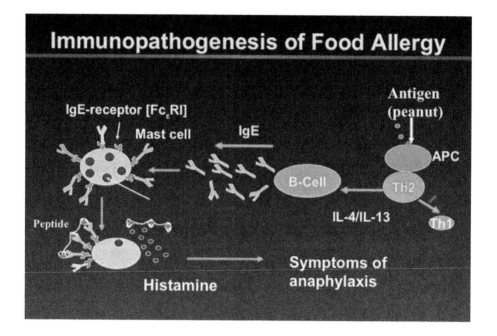

Regulators—and malpractice lawyers—want a good paper trail. As Renata Engler and colleagues put it: "Ultimately, the standard of care will be determined by expert witness testimony in a court of law and is the same for all physicians regardless of whether they use conventional or CAM therapy."[44]

Fair enough. Peanut allergies are too dangerous to subject human beings to a systematic program of food challenges before, during, and after treatment. Even minute amounts of allergen can be fatal, and placebo-controlled trials could be catastrophic. Furthermore, although the allergy epidemic developed through thousands of seemingly random changes in the human immune system over decades, for research, that process had to be compressed into weeks in the lives of test animals.

Thus commenced in 1999 an effort to generate a *murine* model of peanut-induced anaphylaxis—that is, a rodent model, not the stuff you put in sore eyes.[45] There had previously been no completely suitable animal model of peanut allergy to test the efficacy and safety of immunologic therapies.

The standard shortcut, *intraperitoneal* sensitization—direct injection of highly allergenic peanut proteins into the thin, or *serous*, membrane lining the walls of the abdominal and pelvic cavities—was no good. If you're going to model food allergy, it's better to come as close to actual eating as possible. The vision was for an accessible, ingestible botanical treatment, as

32

opposed to a high-priced hospital treatment, with stomach tissue as permeable to the allergens as with naturally occurring food allergies. The alternative chosen was *intragastric* administration—force-feeding doses of peanut antigen and adjuvant.

Tools of the Trade

First, a call went out to the Jackson Laboratory, a publicly supported national repository for mouse models in Bar Harbor, Maine, that was established in 1929. This nonprofit center pioneered the use of inbred laboratory mice to uncover the genetic basis of human development and disease, and today is the site of original research in areas that include cancer, development and aging, immune system and blood disorders, neurological and sensory disorders, and metabolic diseases as well as being the supplier of mice for other laboratories. In 2002, the lab supplied approximately two million mice to the international scientific community.

The process of creating peanut allergy in mice began with an order for five-week-old mice of strain C3H/HeJ, described in the Jackson catalogue as "a general purpose strain in a wide variety of research areas including cancer, immunology, and inflammation, sensorineural, and cardiovascular biology."[46]

Crude extracts of the protein components Ara h1 and Ara h2, which are associated with the most serious allergic reactions more frequently than other components, were created from freshly ground whole peanuts. Cholera toxin was employed as an adjuvant to accelerate the development of allergies—not a small consideration, given the less-than-two-year lifespan of the typical laboratory mouse. Unlike many other bacteria, cholera toxin can resist the highly acidic environment in the stomach. When it arrives in the small intestine, it makes flagella, fibers, that rotate and propel the bacteria corkscrew-like through the mucus of the small intestine.[*,47] Furthermore, a component of cholera toxin has been shown to augment the degranulation of mast cells.[48]

---

* A comparable process takes place in the airways in environments with high levels of airborne "black carbon" from diesel fuels, among other things. The particles penetrate the mucus, allowing exposure to allergens and other irritants, inducing asthma that can be passed on to offspring (http://www.medscape.com/viewarticle/779819).

In tiny concentrations, the toxin makes the tissues more permeable without actually causing cholera or otherwise damaging them.[49] Without this boost, the mucus would perform its normal job of protecting the tissue and would dilute the strength of the peanut allergen. Using the toxin helps bind antigens more tightly to the tissue of the digestive system, where they can essentially bombard the T cells, triggering an immune response disproportionate to the threat. Dr. Li speculates that the strength of the allergic response is a function of the confusion of the innate immune system, which reacts to foreign invaders but lacks memory, and the adaptive system, which has the capacity to learn. As the IgE-equipped mast cells confront the allergens and degranulate, they release histamine and other mediators. Other cells that normally would not be involved in the allergic response perceive a growing emergency and send in "reinforcements." Think of this as Air Force radar confusing a flock of geese with a squadron of enemy airplanes.

A group of mice were left naïve (i.e., with no intervention) to serve as a control. In addition, mice in another control group were fed only the cholera toxin without the peanut antigen. These were "sham-sensitized" mice, which serve as an additional experimental control to ensure that the cholera toxin in the absence of peanut protein did not cause adverse effects in the mice compared to the untreated control. The experimental group was dosed with both cholera toxin and peanut extract.

Each mouse was fed with either 5 mg (equivalent to 1 mg of peanut protein; low dose) or 25 mg (equivalent to 5 mg of peanut protein; high dose) of ground whole peanut together with 10 micrograms of cholera toxin on day one with the initial dose and again on day 7. The low-dose–high-dose experiment was based on an established principle of immunology research, that low doses produce sensitization and high doses produce tolerance. Although the team strongly suspected this dosing strategy would produce the usual results, proving its validity in each particular experiment is part of the protocol.

Three weeks after the initial sensitization, mice were left unfed overnight. The next day, each mouse was challenged intragastrically by having pumped into its stomach 10 mg of crude peanut extract divided into two doses at 30- to 40-minute intervals. Mice surviving the first challenge were rechallenged at week 5. Sham-sensitized mice and naïve mice were challenged in the same manner.

Measuring the Antibodies

Each week, and again one day before challenges, serum samples were drawn from each group of mice after feeding. These samples showed that peanut-specific IgE concentrations increased significantly from week 1 through week 5 in mice sensitized with low-dose peanut (5 mg per mouse) and cholera toxin and from week 2 through week 5 in mice sensitized with high-dose peanut (25 mg per mouse) as well as the toxin; however, levels were significantly higher in the low-dose group than in the high-dose group at both week 3 and week 5, as anticipated.

The First Challenge

Allergen-specific IgE antibodies are not the true measure of allergy. If they were, food allergies could be diagnosed by the numbers. One of the things that makes food allergies so vexing, however, is that an individual may have fairly substantial IgE levels and still not have a clinical allergy. Even the addition of a skin-prick test (SPT), in which a small amount of the offending food is introduced where it may or may not react with the mast cells of the dermis, is not entirely reliable. Short of an oral food challenge, which is not a great screening tool because it may result in a severe reaction, the best allergists rely on an extensive history, which may lead to a diagnosis.

With mice, however, the scruples about inducing anaphylaxis do not apply, so three weeks after the initial sensitization, mice were fed with crude peanut extract at 30- to 40-minute intervals, and the scientists watched.

Within 10 to 15 minutes after the first dose, systemic anaphylactic symptoms started to emerge. The initial symptoms consisted primarily of visible reactions such as puffiness around the eyes and mouth, diarrhea, or both, followed by respiratory reactions, such as wheezing and labored respiration. The most severe reactions were loss of consciousness and death. As expected, the low-dose mice exhibited more severe reactions than those sensitized with the high dose. Fatal or near-fatal anaphylaxis occurred in 12.5% of low-dose–sensitized mice but in none of the high-dose mice. Sham-sensitized—those that received only the cholera toxin and not the peanut—and naïve mice did not show any symptoms of anaphylaxis.

The first measure was observation of "Type 1 hypersensitivity" scored on this scale:

0—no symptoms

1—scratching and rubbing around the nose and head

2—puffiness around the eyes and mouth, *pilar erecti* (hair standing on end), diarrhea, and reduced activity or standing still with an increased respiratory rate

3—wheezing, labored respiration, and cyanosis [blue coloring from loss of oxygen] around the mouth

4—symptoms as in number 3 with loss of consciousness, tremors, and/or convulsion

5—death

The Second Challenge

Two weeks later, the surviving mice were challenged again, resulting in more systemic anaphylactic reactions in both low- and high-dose mice.

One additional finding: A preliminary study had shown no significant anaphylactic reactions if mice were challenged only at week 5; thus, the challenge at week 3 appears to have served as an additional boosting dose. As in the week 3 challenge, symptom scores at the week 5 rechallenge were also significantly higher in the low-dose group than in the high-dose group. The 5-mg-per-mouse dose became the standard for all subsequent studies.

Test Tube Results Confirm Systemic Peanut Allergy and Anaphylaxis Similar to Humans

Skeptics will say quite rightly that people are not the same as animals, the 99% genomic profile notwithstanding. With allergies, however, the mechanisms of a response are quite well understood, and the processes that take place in both species are so similar that direct comparisons can be made both in observation and under the microscope. To understand how comparable they are, a brief look at how allergies happen is in order.

The weapons that our immune systems use to fight certain invaders such as allergens and parasites are housed primarily in effector cells called mast cells and basophils, as mentioned in the first chapter. Antigen-specific IgE attaches itself to high-affinity receptors on the effector cells: mast cells, which mostly lodge in tissues, although some circulate in the blood, and basophils, which only circulate. Mast cells are responsible for the early phases of an allergic reaction because they are present at the site of an exposure, whereas basophils, which take their time getting to the site, account for the late phases, and also encounter allergens that have found their way to other parts of the body. With, say, seasonal allergies, symptoms are generally confined to the area where the allergen is encountered, the sinuses. Part of the inflammatory response is for tissues to swell up and isolate the intense activity. Food allergens present themselves to numerous tissues as they pass from mouth to intestines, however, thus the multiplicity of symptoms, including oral itching and hiving, choking, and diarrhea and vomiting, as well as late-stage symptoms as stray proteins make their way through the blood.

The IgE antibodies look something like lobster claws sticking out from the effector cells and work in pairs. The allergens fit between the claws, forming a bridge, and when they do, the allergic attack begins. The mast cell *degranulates*; that is, it swells up and bursts, and *mediators* are released. When the mast cell's work is done, it's like a piñata after children have pounded it with sticks and all the toys and candy have been unwrapped. The state of the mast cells in the mice and the levels of certain chemicals in the blood would be a telling indicator of how allergic the mice actually were.

Sure enough, the percentage of degranulated mast cells found in the mice's ear tissue was significantly greater in peanut-sensitized mice than in control mice. Plasma histamine levels* were also significantly higher in peanut-sensitized mice than in both sham-sensitized and naïve mice. An additional procedure called a passive cutaneous anaphylaxis (PCA) test was done, in which serum from the blood of one mouse is injected into the skin of another before the antigen challenge. This was done to rule out IgG1-mediated anaphylaxis, in which effector cells are activated through a receptor called FcᵧRIII and can be detected by different biomarkers than IgE reactions. Injection of sera from mice with peanut-allergy–induced reactions elicited a positive PCA reaction following the cutaneous injection of peanut extract, whereas injection of sera from normal wild-type mice did not cause any reaction.

---

* Histamine is a first-responder defense against invading parasites, but when turned on an allergen, it helps cause the itching, sneezing, swelling, and other nasty symtoms of allergies.

In each additional test of T cells, B cells, and various measures of IgE binding, the ways mice responded to allergens in this model resembled human reactions.

Mission accomplished. The researchers had generated a murine model of peanut anaphylaxis. As with humans, these symptoms involved multiple target organs, including the skin, gastrointestinal tract, and respiratory system, with the most severe reactions being fatal. The way was cleared to induce peanut allergy in more mice, measure their reactions in greater detail, and finally, the researchers hoped, test for a cure.

4

A First Test of Efficacy—FAHF-1

O nce the team had developed a reliable method of inducing peanut allergy in mice, it was time to test FAHF-1, the basic nine herbs of WMW with the addition of the magic mushroom *Ling Zhi* and another herb called *Zhi Fu Zi*, which is "used in emergency situations in which there is a complete void of yang energy…characterized by profuse perspiration with clear and cold sweats, intolerance of cold, faint respiration, icy extremities, diarrhea containing undigested food, and faint or imperceptible pulse"[50]—in other words, shock, one of the unmistakable features of full-blown anaphylaxis.

Kamal Srivastava, PhD, who runs the animal studies, joined the team at this point. He says of the process, "At the time much of the animal work was being planned, we met with Dr. Li as a group on a weekly basis. Xiu-Min was very receptive to our suggestions and interpretation of the data, although we needed to have a good argument to convince her."

What followed was, with refinements and variations, a template for more than 10 years of experiments with mice.*[51] For each successive test, the mice would be sensitized using the method already described and then treated—or sham treated—in the same way so that their little bodies would respond in the same ways and provide meaningful apples-to-apples comparisons with each new test.

The identical strain of five-week-old mice—"model" C3H/HeJ—was ordered as in the earlier described experiment to induce allergyalong with the full menu of food and cholera toxin for inducing peanut allergy.

---

* All experimental data in this chapter is drawn from the same article.

Components of Herbal Medicines in FAHF-1

	TCM Materia Medica (pinyin)	Equivalent pharmaceutical name	Amount (g)	Part used
1	Wu mei	Fructus pruni mume	30	Fruit
2	Ling zhi (Chi)	Ganoderma lucidum	15	Fruiting body
3	Fu zi (zhi)	Radix lateralis aconiti carmichaeli praeparata	3	Root
4	Chuan jiao	Pericarpium zanthoxyli bungeani	1.5	Seed
5	Xi xin	Herba cum radice asari	1	Whole
6	Huang lian (Chuan)	Rhizoma coptidis	9	Root
7	Huang bai	Cortex phellodendri	6	Root
8	Gan jiang	Rhizoma zingiberis officinalis	6	Root
9	Gui zhi	Ramulus cinnamomi cassiae	3	Twig
10	Ren shen (Hong)	Radix ginseng	9	Root
11	Dang gui (shen)	Corpus radix angelicae sinensis	9	Root

All of the herbal medicines were ordered from the China Academy of Traditional Chinese Medicine Sciences, Xiyuan Chinese Medicine Research and Pharmaceutical Manufacturer in Beijing, and inspected by pharmacists according to the Chinese Herbal Medicine Materia Medica and Pharmacopoeia of the People's Republic of China at the China–Japan Friendship Hospital, Beijing, China. This supplier has been used throughout the process to ensure uniformity and accountability. Each big hospital in China has its own pharmaceutical manufacturing facilities that make all the preparations used there, right down to saline solution. Although this might someday be a problem for supplying the export market for particular herbal-based drugs if demand picks up, for experimental purposes, this is not an issue; however, all medications imported undergo further quality-control testing at Mount Sinai.

FAHF-1 Preparation

This section should be read carefully by anyone who envisions do-it-yourself treatment from herbs ordered through the Internet or purchased at an apothecary in Chinatown. Imagine doing the following every day for months at a time!

The daily human adult dosage, based on figures in the Pharmacopeia of the People's Republic of China, was 92.5 grams (a little less than 4 ounces) of raw herbs, *decocted* (water-extracted). To begin, *Ling zhi* and *Zhi Fu Zi* were boiled individually for 2 hours, and the decoction was filtered and *lyophilized*, or freeze dried, and the remaining components—*Wu mei, Chuan jiao, Xi xin, Huang lian, Huang bai, Gan jiang, Gui zhi, Ren shen, Dang gui*—were then added and boiled for an additional 1 hour. After lyophilizing and mixing, the yield was 15 grams of dried extract—about half an ounce. Then, using conversion table based on body surface area from another Chinese text, *Pharmacology for Experimental Studies*, a dose of 21 milligrams of freeze-dried FAHF-1 in 0.5 mL of water was administered to each mouse twice daily.

Two groups of mice were sensitized with 5 mg of peanut plus 10 micrograms of cholera toxin, administered intragastrically and boosted 1 and 3 weeks later. One week after the final sensitization dose, some of these mice were treated, receiving 21 mg of FAHF-1 or being sham-treated with water, administered by intragastric gavage twice daily for 7 weeks.

Then came the challenge for all three groups—10 mg of crude peanut extract administered intragastrically. Naïve mice served as additional controls.

Plasma was collected 30 minutes after challenge, and histamine levels were determined through use of an enzyme immunoassay kit made by a French company, which I only mention because I am intrigued by the global supply chain for science. Degranulated mast cells in ear tissues were counted in samples collected 40 minutes after the peanut challenge.

Peanut-specific serum IgE concentrations were measured along with total serum IgG and IgA. Splenocytes—cells that originate in the spleen, including T and B lymphocytes, dendritic cells and macrophages, which have different immune functions—were taken from 5 mice in each group for culture and study. Sera from treated peanut-allergic mice were obtained one day before challenge and subjected to biochemical analyses of liver- and kidney-function testing. Toxicity was measured, which was a crucial step when working with this particular set of herbs because, as was mentioned briefly earlier, a couple of the herbs did raise red flags.

Starting 30 to 40 minutes after the challenge, anaphylactic symptoms were scored.

In the sham-treated group—the ones that received the placebo—80% exhibited symptoms such as itching (score 1; 10%); puffiness around the eyes, swelling around the mouth, and diarrhea (score 2; 30%); labored respiration (score 3; 20%); and loss of consciousness or little activity after prodding (score 4; 20%). This list alone should make us grateful that mice make such effective stand-ins for people for such research. By contrast, FAHF-1–treated mice and naïve mice exhibited no symptoms after challenge.

During anaphylaxis, one of the most dangerous effects is a collapse in blood pressure, which is accompanied by lower temperatures as the heart labors to delivery blood to vital organs and extremities. This indicator should make anyone who has ever taken care of a sick child even more pleased that mice make such apt research subjects. Each mouse had its temperature taken rectally 30 minutes after the peanut challenge. Just in case you were curious about how such an undignified procedure is administered to a mouse, a ¾ inch (19 mm) long probe with a ball tip 1.7 mm (0.07 inches) in diameter attached to a 5-foot cable attached to a computer.

By every measure, the results were encouraging. Core body temperatures showed substantial drops among the sham-treated mice, with little difference in the naïve group and the FAHF-1 treated mice.

Blood assays, too, supported the observed results.

Tissues of the sham-treated mice revealed the remains of many degranulated mast cells after the challenge, while those that had been treated showed levels not significantly above the sham group. Plasma histamine levels also were markedly elevated in the sham-treated group but not in the FAHF-1–treated group. The naïve mice had the lowest levels all.

Peanut IgE tracked these other numbers closely. When FAHF-1 treatment was initiated four weeks after sensitization, peanut-specific IgE levels were significantly higher in both sensitized groups than in the naïve group.

No more mice were sacrificed and no more treatment given, but IgE was monitored in the survivors for an additional four weeks. At the end of that time, levels were essentially the same as they had been when treatment was discontinued and were roughly half those for the sham-treated mice.

Finally, T cells from sham-treated mice produced much higher levels of the cytokines associated with allergic responses.

This was a grand slam for FAHF-1, and it was achieved with no detectable toxicity, a prerequisite for eventual approval. "First do no harm" is a part of the process.

The discussion at the end of the published article draws some interesting inferences from the results that can only excite peanut-allergy families everywhere:

> In this study, we treated PN-sensitized mice with an herbal formulation and demonstrated that this treatment abrogated PN-induced anaphylactic symptoms and significantly reduced PN-specific serum IgE levels. Our results suggest that an immune system already "committed" to an anaphylactic pathway can be normalized, at least partially, after treatment with FAHF-1 in this model. (p. 644)

They demonstrated that the herbal formula suppressed production of Th2 cytokines, the ones associated with allergies, and speculated that it directly inhibited allergen-induced B-cell activation, "thereby reducing the number of allergen-specific molecules bound to mast cells."

Moreover—and this is very important for anyone who worries that reduced Th2, allergy-associated activity may also compromise acquired immunity to, say, polio—Th1 activity, which controls immunity to infectious disease, was unaffected.

If that is the case, that Th2 activity is reduced while Th1 is not, it means that fewer "battle-ready allergy troops" will be out there looking for a fight when the enemy—peanut proteins—present themselves with no detrimental effects for the body's ability to fight infection. The researchers also observed that the herbal formula may reduce intestinal permeability, meaning that fewer proteins will have access to the bloodstream, which is the vehicle for delivering allergens to the multiple organ systems whose activation defines anaphylaxis.

The paper ends on the cautious note that is frustrating to people desperate for treatment: "Although animal models are not identical to human disease and further studies regarding effects of long-term administration and/or interactions with prescription drugs are required, this study suggests that FAHF-1 might be useful for the treatment of PN allergy and perhaps of other IgE-mediated food allergies." (p. 645)

The results were good. Very good.

5

Process of Elimination

F or the next phase, two herbs were eliminated from FAHF-1—*Zhi Fu Zi* and *Xi Xin* (*Herba Asari*). Both are useful, like *Ling Zhi*, for treating shock.

This decision was made for several reasons. The active ingredients in these herbs are alkaloids, which means they are in a class of drugs that includes cocaine, morphine, and caffeine. This is not to imply "guilt by association," but alkaloids are tricky to use in refined forms. As you will read, refining would be imperative in the effort to turn the basic formula into manageable medication.

A better-known example of a TCM ingredient containing alkaloids that doesn't make an easy transition from its herbal state to a refined form is *ma huang*, which has been used by TCM practitioners to treat asthma and other conditions for thousands of years. It was highly valued in ancient China and environs, and it has been found in tombs along with other treasures.

The active ingredient in *ma huang* is ephedra, which in its synthetic version was taken orally for asthma by the early 20th century in the United States.[52] (Safe asthma treatments were hard to come by in those days: "asthma cigarettes" made from the leaves of *datura stramonium*, also known as jimpson weed, a hallucinogen, were the only other remedy in common use.[53]) More recently, ephedra was legally used as a diet aid (at much higher concentrations than for asthma), but it was linked to sudden death from ephedrine toxicity, nephrolithiasis, and acute hepatitis and is now banned. It is also an ingredient in the decongestant pseudoephedrine and its rogue cousin, methamphetamine.

Both *Zhi Fu Zi* and *Xi Xin* raised questions with the US Food and Drug Administration (FDA) because of quality-control issues, enunciated at length in a 2000 publication of Guidance for Industry for botanicals.[54] The FDA was concerned about residual aconitine ("a poisonous solid that occurs naturally in the roots and leaves of aconite plants such as monkshood and wolfsbane"[55]).* The scientific name of *Zhi Fu Zi (Radix Lateralis **Aconiti** Carmichaeli Praeparata)* leaves nothing to the imagination on this score.

Xi Xin was the subject of a 2001 warning on botanicals that contain aristolochic acid, which had been detected in numerous samples imported into the United States and in Europe, and was associated with kidney failure. "The ingredient will only be allowed to enter the U.S. when adequate testing shows that the suspect ingredients are free of aristolochic acid."[56] *Aristolochia clematitis*, or European bloodwort, was the subject of an 2013 *New Yorker* article called "Poisoned Land." The author, Elif Batuman, says that he and his father, a kidney specialist, visited a lab that had 400 kidneys in bottles, and that his dad said he had never seen kidneys so badly shrunken. The degree of toxicity may vary according to the soil composition of particular regions where these herbs are grown.

Fortunately, based on their reading of the TCM formulation system, the team determined that neither *Zhi Fu Zi* nor *Xi Xin* was crucial to the long-term therapeutic goals of their research. If they had been, it might have been worth the time and expense of ensuring toxin-free supplies; however, the shock-protection qualities of *Zhi Fu Zi* could be achieved through "magic mushroom." *Xi Xin* primarily helped relieve stomach pain, so the researchers increased the dose of *Gan Jiang* (gingerroot) which is safe and accomplishes the same thing.

As mentioned earlier, one big challenge was to find a reliable supply of *Ling Zhi* with the requisite degree of purity for manufacture. With the help of a university professor friend, Dr. Li did manage to locate a remote, undeveloped forest where the mushroom grows wild. They compared samples from eight other regions, some of them quite close to this particular forest, and found those samples wanting.

---

* Fans of horror movies will recall that wolfsbane was used to cure people afflicted with lycanthropy—werewolves.

When food-allergy moms ask me why versions of one FAHF or another aren't widely available, seeing as how versions of them have been in use for centuries, this is the kind of thing I tell them. You can't mix these things at home out of things you find at your health-food store. Even if they were all safe, different parts of the plant are used for the different ingredients—whole fruit, seeds, roots, or twigs depending on where the active ingredients are concentrated. This is not a job for amateurs.

I also found the extent of regulatory coverage very impressive. Alternative medicine may get some slack in the gray area between supplements and medicines, but at least in this instance, government scientists are doing their job in protecting us from known adulterants. Chemists led by Dr. Nan Yang, a six-year veteran of Dr. Li's team, are responsible for, among other things, ensuring quality and purity of all medicines and extracts used in their research. The lab adheres to European standards, which are, in fact, even higher than American ones. Each new batch received from China is compared to previous ones that have been certified free of pesticides, heavy metals, and other contaminants.

The chemistry also involves isolation of active ingredients, "fingerprinting" them, studying their pharmacokinetics (what the body does to the drug, as opposed to what the drug does to the body, which is called pharmacodynamics, as defined by wikipedia,) and monitoring absorption, first in cell lines, then in mice, and eventually in human subjects. Eventually, as they continue to isolate the active ingredients, they may be able to assemble these compounds in the laboratory, but for now, we must depend on the unique combinations provided by nature.

6

Proof

In 2005, Dr. Li's team published the first of two landmark studies signaling the efficacy of FAHF-2. The title of the first of these, led by Kamal D. Srivastava, who directs biological studies for the Sinai team, states the case very directly: "The Chinese Herbal Medicine Formula FAHF-2 Completely Blocks Anaphylactic Reactions in a Murine Model of Peanut Allergy." This study included data from a series of five experiments over a period of two and a half years.[57]

The procedure was always the same. After sensitization, with boosting at 5 weeks and 7 weeks, and with sham and naïve mice as controls, all mice were challenged with ground peanut at week 10 (one week post therapy). To determine whether FAHF-2 protected against anaphylaxis for a significant period of time after therapy, mice received 6 sensitization doses at weekly intervals, followed by boosting doses at weeks 6 and 8. Mice were challenged at week 12 or 14 (3 and 5 weeks post therapy). An earlier study showed that 6 weeks after the week-8 boost was the latest time at which mice still exhibited hypersensitivity to initial challenge.

The mice were assessed for systemic anaphylaxis signs, temperature, and plasma histamine levels. In addition, immediately before the second intragastric peanut challenge, two mice from each group were injected with blue dye and their footpads were examined for blue color that would indicate leakage from the capillaries—indicative of the drastically lower blood pressure that is a symptom of anaphylaxis. (Many homeowners may be familiar with this phenomenon if they rely on circulating hot water to heat their homes. In the event that the pump fails, the solder seals in the pipes may start to leak as water pressure falls. I speak from experience.)

Incidence of Anaphylactic Reactions
(across multiple experiments over 2.5 years)

	Challenge time	Sham		FAHF-2		Naive	
		n/total	Anaphylactic score Median (Range)	n/total	Anaphylactic score (Median)	n/total	Anaphylactic score (Median)
Exp.# 1	W 10	9/9	3 (2-4)	0/9	0***	0/9	0
Exp.# 2	W12	8/8	3 (2-4)	0/4	0***	0/5	0
Exp.# 3	W14	8/8	3 (2-3)	0/4	0**	0/5	0
Exp.# 4	W14	8/8	3 (2-4)	0/4	0***	0/5	0
Exp.# 5	W14	5/5	3 (2-3)	0/5	0***	0/5	0
Totals		38/38	3 (2-4)	0/26	0###	0/29	0

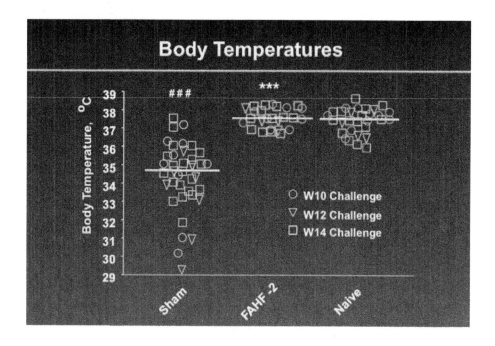

Body Temperatures

○ W10 Challenge
▽ W12 Challenge
□ W14 Challenge

48

The results were dramatic. After challenge at week 10 (1 week post therapy), all sham-treated mice developed anaphylactic reactions, with a median score of 3. In contrast, FAHF-2–treated mice exhibited no anaphylactic signs. The same results were found after week-12 and -14 challenges.

Dr. Sampson asked that the experiment be repeated, and it was done five times, all told, over a two-and-a-half-year period. The pooled data show that all 38 sham-treated mice developed anaphylaxis, with a median anaphylactic score of 3, indicating a severe anaphylactic reaction. In contrast, none of the 26 FAHF-2–treated mice and none of 29 naïve mice developed anaphylaxis after challenge. These results demonstrated that FAHF-2 "has potent protective properties" against peanut-induced anaphylaxis and that the complete protection was consistent and relatively persistent. Plasma histamine and IgE levels were all consistent with efficacy of FAHF-2.

Just as dramatic were the figures for loss of body temperature. Mouse normal, just above 37 degrees Celsius, is essentially the same as human normal. For all the challenges in all experiments, the median loss of temperature was more than two degrees Celsius (to 95° Fahrenheit) for the sham-treated mice, which is essentially the lower limit for normal metabolism and bodily function.[58] Those for the treated and naïve groups were normal.

Meanwhile, the feet of the sham-treated mice showed a distinct blue tint from capillary leakage, while the FAHF-2 mice were indistinguishable from the naïve.

In 2007, Dr. Li and a team of four other researchers published the second of these watershed critical studies, titled "Induction of Tolerance after Establishment of Peanut Allergy by the Food Allergy Herbal Formula-2 Is Associated with Up-Regulation of Interferon-g."[59] Interferon-gamma (IFN-g) is a cytokine with known anti-allergenic properties, secreted by the Th1 helper cells. Up-regulation is a good thing for reducing the severity of the allergic response; the greater the output of the Th1 cells compared to Th2, the less allergic the patient will be.

The article also provides another glimpse of the continually fascinating—to me, anyway—commercial supply chain that supports laboratory research. This work can't be done with materials from your local pet shop, pharmacy, and hardware stores. All procedures and the paraphernalia

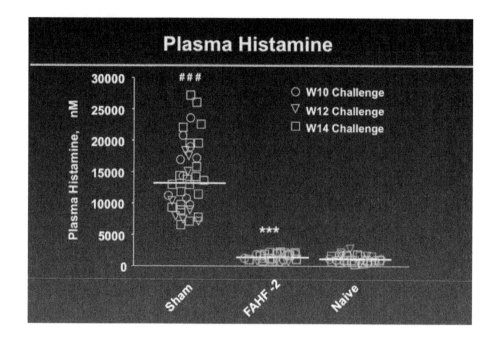

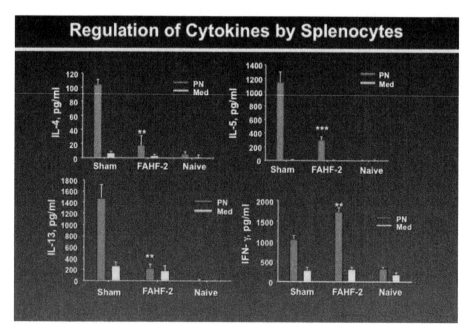

required to perform them are documented in the peer-reviewed article. If the proof of an experiment is that it must be replicable, following this template, you should be able to do the same thing at home, if you have the requisite thousands of dollars of equipment and skills.

Once again, an order went out to Jackson Labs.

The rest of the inventory included freshly ground whole roasted peanut and crude peanut extract (CPE), cholera toxin. There were also numerous pieces of specialized apparatus.

An ample supply of FAHF-2 formula was secured from a certified medical herb facility in Beijing and its quality controlled according to the standards of Pharmacopoeia of China.

Blood samples were obtained from tail veins before sensitization began and throughout the process. Sera were collected and stored at –80° Celsius (–176° Fahrenheit) until analyzed to determine levels of peanut-specific IgE, which indicates sensitization to allergens. These would provide snapshots of changes in immune activity along the way.

As before, after a peanut-free diet for the first 5 weeks of their lives, some of the mice were initiated into a crash course of life-threatening allergies while a control group of mice were left naïve (not given peanuts at all). For the peanut group, normal food was supplemented with 10 mg of ground peanuts weekly for 5 weeks, with subsequent boosting at the rate of 50 mg—all delivered directly into the stomach via a feeding tube.

After completing the week-8 boosting protocol, 8 mice—4 naïve and 4 peanut-sensitized—were given an extra-large dose of peanut (200 mg) and then observed.

After 30 minutes, 3 of the sensitized mice had 2 symptoms, and the 4th had 3 symptoms, while the naïve mice had none. All 4 allergic mice had subnormal body temperature, while the nonallergic ones were all normal. The blood showed, sure enough, plasma histamine levels at combat strength in the highly allergic mice. Serum peanut-specific IgE levels—the antibodies primed for the appearance of peanut proteins—had also been high. This indicated that T-cell activity had created an imbalance between Th1 and Th2. Greater Th2 output had skewed the immune system toward allergic activity.

Clearly, the sensitized mice had been highly allergic and the naïve mice had not.

Time to Commence Treatment

FAHF-2 was administered intragastrically twice daily for 7 weeks. An additional group of peanut-allergic mice received only an equal amount of water (sham treatment). Finally, the naïve mice served as controls. All mice received peanut challenges (200 mg/mouse) 24 hours after the completion of therapy at week 14 and again 4 weeks later. Cholera toxin as a mucosal adjuvant was coadministered with peanut at all times except during the final challenge. Anaphylactic-reaction scores and body temperatures were determined approximately 30 minutes following each challenge. Immediately following the final peanut challenge and evaluation of reactions, mice were killed and lymphocytes from the spleen and lymph nodes were isolated for study.[60]

Although these cells can survive for a time outside the host, the numbers that circulate in the blood are not sufficient for test-tube research, so, using a method employed by British researchers,[61] the team cloned the lymphocytes collected from the blood of each group until they had a workable concentration. The team then separated the lymphocytes into *aliquots*—identical small portions—allowing for precise comparison of uniform samples.

These were cultured with peanut antigen to show which ones would produce Th1-IFN-g cytokines indicating immunity or Th2 interleukins indicating allergy.

Finally, all the observed results and numbers were analyzed according to various standard methods.

The data were unambiguous. Peanut-hypersensitive mice that received FAHF-2 treatment were completely protected against anaphylactic reactions following the challenge, and their body temperatures were in the normal range, whereas all sham-treated mice exhibited anaphylactic reactions and had core body temperatures significantly lower than those of naïve mice. And, unlike as in corticosteroid therapy, there was no evidence of reduced immunity to infections. As Dr. Engler points out: "This is what is so profoundly new about this therapy—a steroid-like action against allergic inflammation without compromising infection defense *and* persistence of the effect, in contrast to steroid, where tapering is associated with the problem flaring again."

All sham-treated mice continued to develop anaphylactic reactions following the second post-therapy challenge at week 18, whereas no anaphylactic reactions were observed in those treated with FAHF-2–treated mice. These results demonstrated that FAHF-2–established tolerance persisted for at least 4 weeks after therapy.

The observed results were borne out by the laboratory findings. FAHF-2 treatment suppressed histamine release in peanut-allergic mice. Plasma histamine levels were markedly elevated in all peanut-sensitized, sham-treated mice at week 14 following peanut challenge, while treated sensitized mice had significantly lower histamine levels effectively indistinguishable from those of naïve mice following both post-therapy challenges.

FAHF-2 also reduced peanut-specific IgE levels and increased peanut-specific IgG2a levels in peanut-allergic mice. Again, like IgG4 in humans, IgG2a is a "blocking antibody" that prevents allergens from triggering an allergic reaction. These antibodies compete with IgE for receptor space on effector cells, either mast cells or basophils. As Th2 activity diminishes, a higher proportion of IgG antibodies occupy the available mast cell openings. With a half-life of just two days, the disenfranchised IgE antibodies circulating in the blood have a brief shot at finding a perch.

The short half-life of serum IgE is important because it accounts for the unreliability of blood IgE tests. Children with no history of allergy can show high allergen-specific IgE levels as measured by a radioallergosorbent test [RAST], sending their parents into a panic. The circulating IgE antibodies can't do any damage unless they have attached themselves to effector cells, however. Once the antibodies find a place to hang their hats (i.e., on a mast cell or a basophil) they have a half-life of 6 to 8 weeks, which makes them a threat for triggering a reaction when the right allergen comes along. SPTs are more reliable than RAST because the IgE is situated on the mast cells in the skin and will prompt a local reaction.[62] SPTs are relatively safe because the skin is isolated from the blood stream, so a skin reaction will only rarely spread from the skin and involve other organ systems in an anaphylactic reaction. Anaphylaxis is generally defined as an allergic reaction in two or more organ systems, such as the skin, the digestive tract, and, most dangerously, the airways.

Before treatment (week 8), all peanut-sensitized mice had similar peanut-specific IgE levels. After treatment, however, these levels were significantly reduced. At the time of first post-challenge (week 14) measurement, treated mice showed much lower IgE than did the sham-treated mice, and the level remained significantly lower 4 weeks later (week 18). In fact, the reduction appeared more pronounced at week 18 than at week 14, demonstrating persistent suppression of IgE production. Keep in mind that the life expectancy of a lab mouse is two years. If the same level of protection holds true for humans, each 4-week period would amount to about 3 years.

IgG2a levels were significantly higher in FAHF-2–treated allergic mice compared with sham-treated allergic mice following 2 weeks of FAHF-2 treatment (week 10) and remained significantly higher up to 4 weeks after therapy was complete (week 18), indicating that FAHF-2 also had a persistent effect on IgG2a production.

The Effect on T-helper Cells

The next step was to measure the effect of FAHF-2 on cytokine profiles. Clearly, FAHF-2 seemed to be effective, but why? What effects on the various proteins appear to be involved in establishing efficacy? It's a bit like taking a census; an urban planner may note changes in the life of a city—changing crime rates in different neighborhoods, school enrollments rising and falling, fire alarms, both real and false—but there's nothing like a census to understand what lies behind the changes. Likewise, it's not enough to show that a treatment like FAHF-2 works. You have to know why. What are the specific mechanisms by which it heals? What clues lie in the cell counts that might point to further improvements in the formula, and also what complications?

In a healthy immune system, there is equilibrium between Th1 activity and Th2. As I explained earlier, with allergies, there is disproportionate Th2 output, resulting in excessive IgE—ten times or more normal levels in a very allergic person. With autoimmune disorders, the imbalance tips the other way. The body essentially loses tolerance to some of its own tissues and attacks them as if they were foreign.[63]

The same disproportion of Th2 activity pertains with all allergies, not just food. That is why research on the body chemistry of allergic rhinitis and asthma can help explain the action of FAHF-2 on food allergies as well.

In a 2009 article on her work with asthma treatment, Dr. Li and her coauthor wrote:

> T_H1 and T_H2 responses are felt to be mutually antagonistic, such that they normally exist in equilibrium and cross-regulate each other. An optimum T_H1-T_H2 balance has been suggested as necessary to maintain healthy immune homeostasis. Loss of such balance has been hypothesized to underlie allergic asthma through a shift in immune responses from a T_H1 *(IFN-γ)* pattern toward a T_H2 *(IL-4, IL-5, and IL-13)* profile, which promotes IgE production; eosinophilic inflammation, activation, and survival; and enhanced airway smooth muscle contractility.[64] (p. 301)

One established method of determining the prevalence of Th1 and Th2 activity is to harvest and culture cells from organs where large numbers of these lymphocytes are created. The spleen, which produces *splenocytes*, and the *mesenteric lymph nodes*, which produce MLN cells, are rich sources for gathering these cells. An abundance of the cytokines IL-4, IL-5, and IL-13, all interleukins, would show more activity by Th2 cells associated with allergies. More interferon gamma, or IFN-γ, and TGF-β (transforming growth factor beta, which controls proliferation, cellular differentiation, and other functions in most cells, as well as IL-10 levels) would indicate greater Th1 activity.

As predicted, MLN cells and splenocytes from FAHF-2–treated mice produced significantly less IL-4, IL-5, and IL-13 than their counterparts from sham-treated mice. MLN cells and splenocytes from FAHF-2–treated mice produced significantly greater amounts of IFN-γ.

No differences in TGF-β production were detected in FAHF-2–treated mice when compared with the sham-treated group, whereas small but significant decreases were observed in IL-10 levels. The most pronounced effect of FAHF-2 on Th1 and Th2 responses was on MLN cells in which IFN-γ production was increased up to tenfold. This finding was consistent in two separate experiments.

At this point, I must tell readers that if they are frustrated by the continual addition of new terminology, particularly that created by the accretion of letters, some in Greek and some in English, and numbers, I share your discontents. These appear from nowhere in successive published articles as we get deeper into the biochemistry. In conversations with MDs, I found that when these individuals are not specially trained in immunology, there's no special reason for them to know what I am talking about either.

Interpreting the Data

At this stage in an experiment, the researchers sit down and analyze what has been proven, what has not, and what remains to be done. In this study, they "found that FAHF-2 treatment initiated when hypersensitivity was fully established completely protected peanut-allergic mice from anaphylaxis, and that this protection persisted for at least 4 weeks after discontinuing therapy." The "results indicated that FAHF-2 *may* prove to be of therapeutic value for peanut-allergic patients" (emphasis added) More studies would explore how long this protective effect persists. Qu et al 853

On key measures, FAHF-2 treatment was shown to have completely blocked histamine release, which was consistent with FAHF-2's prevention of anaphylactic reactions. The researchers found that peanut-specific IgE levels began to decline about 2 weeks after treatment began and were significantly reduced immediately after completing treatment (week 14). These levels remained significantly depressed 4 weeks after therapy ceased (week 18) as compared with sham treatment, suggesting that suppressed peanut-specific IgE production may be associated with protection against peanut anaphylaxis. Interestingly, although FAHF-2 treatment did not eliminate peanut-specific IgE, it still produced complete clinical protection against anaphylaxis and completely blocked histamine release. "Therefore, the protective effect of FAHF-2 in peanut-induced anaphylaxis cannot be explained solely by the reduction of peanut-specific IgE." Qu et al 853

Several mechanisms appear to play additional roles in the FAHF-2 protective effect. Levels of IgG2a were increased significantly beginning 2 weeks after treatment was initiated. That was before peanut-specific IgE began to fall, and the IgG2a levels remained significantly elevated up to 4 weeks post therapy. "Thus, the enhancement of peanut-specific IgG2a levels also may be involved in protecting peanut-allergic mice from anaphylactic reactions." FAHF-2 protection may also be associated with its effect on other effector cells such as mast cells and basophils. This possibility suggested further experiments. Qu et al 853

There's something both exhilarating and annoying about studies like this one. The exhilaration stems from the promising results. For something as mysterious as a life-threatening allergy to "America's food"—the peanut and all its derivatives—the prospect of a cure is tantalizing. Moreover, the idea that the counter-magic can be proven not only in the achievement of tolerance but also by counting cells and assaying biochemistry leads us to hope. But evidence does not make for unequivocal assertions of victory. The results are only promising. The mouse results must be hedged—this *may* work. More work lies ahead.

7

Whole Greater Than the Sum of Its Parts

When a compound containing many ingredients is shown to be effective, science demands that its parts be tested to show whether one or more can achieve a comparable result. Each ingredient you can drop from the final product reduces complexity and the expense of eventual manufacture. The Mount Sinai team did a study published in 2008[65] to test each herb using the same strain of mice, sensitization, and challenge protocols as the complete FAHF-2. However, the presence of an individual component may be crucial not for what it does in and of itself, but by increasing the bioavailability (effective absorption) of another—that is, the effective absorption of an active compound—or individual components may influence different pathways individually but unlock a productive response only together.

Phellodendron chinense achieved the best results with three of four mice; however, no individual herb treatment reproduced the broad-based immunological effects of FAHF-2, including suppression of IgE and the Th2 cytokines that signal its production, and elevation of the Th1, which produces the beneficial IFN-γ and antibody IgG2a. Some individual herbs appeared to suppress peanut-stimulated-Th2 cytokine production in splenocytes.

For example, *Phellodendron chinense* treatment appeared to suppress Th2 cytokines IL-4 and perhaps IL-13, but not IL-5, whereas *Angelica sinensis* and *Panax ginseng* treatment appeared to decrease two of the three. *Phellodendron chinense*, although the most effective single herb overall, was insufficient as a stand-alone treatment. In later experiments, *Phellodendron chinense* lost its effectiveness over repeated peanut challenges, in contrast to FAHF-2, which protected against anaphylaxis in several challenges over 6 months.

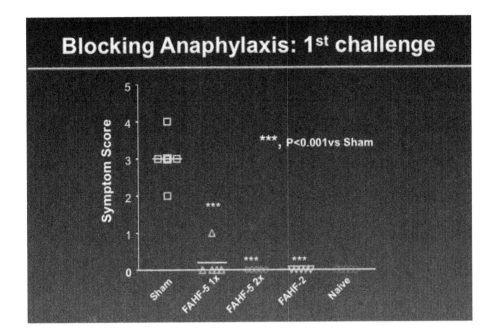

Because no single herb was effective, a simplified food allergy herbal Formula (sFAHF), which included *Phellodendron chinense, Zingiber officinalis,* and *Ganoderma lucidum*, was also investigated. These three herbs collectively showed the most favorable responses in protection from anaphylaxis, suppression of IgE, and modulation of Th2/Th1 cytokines, presenting a potentially simpler alternative to FAHF-2; however, sFAHF prevented anaphylactic symptoms in only 3 of 5 mice, and plasma histamine levels were not significantly reduced after challenge.

After analyzing all 10 herbs in this way, the authors concluded, "Taken together the results suggest that all the herbs of FAHF-2 are likely required for the ability to provide complete and lasting protection against anaphylaxis and alter Th2/Th1 immune responses in a manner beneficial for therapy of food allergy." p. 658

More on the Magic in the "Magic Mushroom"

This science is not necessarily sequential. Although clinical investigations proceed in a careful stepwise manner to avoid unnecessary harm to patients, other aspects of the science, particularly delving into the mechanisms behind the effects, can be investigated by whoever has a hypothesis worth testing and the funds to do it. Dr. Li's group knew that some substances in the mushroom *Ling Zhi* are potentially bioactive (such as the steroid-related substances called triterpenes), but which ones were important in the mushroom's anti-allergy properties? They explored this question in a paper (unpublished as of this writing) with the evocative title "Ganoderic Acid C1 Isolated from *Ganoderma lucidum* Suppresses Macrophage and Human Peripheral Blood Mononuclear Cell TNF-α Production by Down-Regulating MAPK, NF-κB and AP-1 Signaling Pathways."[66]

Noting that *Ganoderma lucidum* had been used for thousands of years because of its "broad beneficial pharmacological actions," they were particularly drawn to an association with inhibiting production of TNF-a (tumor necrosis factor-alpha). They noted, "TNF-α plays a key role in the immediate host defense against invading microorganisms prior to activation of the adaptive immune system. Excessive levels of TNF-α have been implicated in mediating or exacerbating a number of diseases including Alzheimer's disease, cancer, major depression, and refractory inflammatory diseases including Crohn's disease, rheumatoid arthritis, and asthma."

Dr. Li's team hypothesized that the triterpenes—the compounds in the mushroom that impart a bitter taste—were involved in the inhibition of TNF-α. They have started testing this by first isolating various compounds from *Ling Zhi* and then determining which ones can inhibit TNF-α production by white blood cells isolated from patients with asthma and Crohn's disease (more on TNF-α and Crohn's disease appears in the chapter "Beyond Food Allergies."). Extracts containing mainly triterpenes proved potent inhibitors of TNF-α production by macrophages, the most powerful of which appears to be ganoderic acid C1 (GAC1). The potency also depends on the amount used. It has the advantage of also being non-toxic. These results, which mimicked the effects of the whole mushroom extract, lend credence to the team's hypothesis that triterpenes are the active substance.

8

How Long Does It Last?

Among the food-allergy parents with whom I interact regularly through social media, there are several, for want of a better word, *factions*. One of these consists of mothers who have sought out OIT outside of clinical trials despite the fact that it is not approved for general treatment. OIT is available as part of continuing academic study, which is free, although it often involves considerable expense and travel time to arrive at the participating teaching hospitals. Places in the trials are limited and available only to those who meet certain health criteria. A number of doctors in private practice administer this treatment from protocols that have been proven to their personal satisfaction but are not cleared by the FDA for clinical use. Families usually pay cash, although there are more reports of insurance companies picking up some of the tab, and they often travel hundreds or sometimes thousands of miles to see these doctors.

As a father, I sympathize with parents who are choosing some relief from fear for their children's health even if the outcomes are still unproven to a regulatory standard. Much is unsettled, particularly if the result requires perpetual maintenance dosing. As I can attest to personally, a daily handful of peanuts or Peanut M&Ms sounds better than Grandpa's Lipitor, but I believe that as these mostly very young patients grow up, they will tire of maintenance dosing. Many who grow up under the threat of anaphylaxis to a particular food never develop a taste for it, which means they must continue to find creative ways to take their medicine *forever*. And then there's the common bane of allergic and asthmatic existence, which is to equate absence of symptoms with cure; people who aren't symptomatic for long periods of time get careless. Although it is still too early to say definitively, it seems to me that children who undergo OIT are good candidates to tempt fate as teenagers. Dr. Robert Wood of Johns Hopkins attracted a great deal of attention at the 2013 meeting of the American Academy of Allergy Asthma and Immunology when he announced that desensitization to milk wasn't holding up after 3 to 5 years. He said, "Some of the more dramatic failures had looked like absolute successes in the study. They were tolerating huge amounts of milk; they were about as close to 'cured' as we could imagine."[67] Finally, there is the generic problem of all chronic disease management—patients just stop taking their medicine.

For all these reasons, the prospect of a permanent cure, or at least long-lasting protection, becomes very attractive, which raises the stakes for FAHF-2's success.

We saw in the first phase of Dr. Li's mouse research that protection persisted for as long as 5 weeks past the end of treatment.[68] How much further could it go, and what would it reveal about the mechanisms that produced the improvement? Would its effects go beyond reducing allergies and lead to overall suppression of the immune system, which is the problem with oral and injectable corticosteroids? Such corticosteroids reduce inflammation, which can save lives in an emergency (or make it possible for a stricken athlete to return to the lineup), but regular use leaves the body vulnerable to opportunistic infections and other rebound effects.[69]

An unbalanced therapy could create other problems as well, leaving patients vulnerable to attacks from within their own bodies. Could it cause cancer, for example? This was a red flag raised in the early use of the anti-IgE antibody omalizumab, although that has largely been discredited. (Xolair remains, however, painful to pay for and painful to receive and can be allergenic in its own right for some.) And as mentioned, if a treatment reduced IgE but increased IgG excessively, it could result in some form of autoimmune disease.

The desired outcome was immunomodulation. That is, IgE[vil] production would go down but not disappear, and the production of IgG[ood] would increase without taking over completely.

The first experiment with FAHF-2 treatment had shown that tolerance to peanut for 4 weeks after therapy was associated with increased production of the IFN-γ cytokines by CD8+ T cells, which in turn correlates with protection from anaphylaxis.

TGF-β, a protein that controls proliferation, cellular differentiation, and other functions in most cells,[70] was not affected. TGF-β also plays a part in a range of diseases including cancer, allaying concern that recalibrating the immune system in one way might unbalance it in another. There was a slight but significant reduction of IL-10 production as well. These findings suggested that FAHF-2 might have a long-lasting effect and that increased IFN-γ output by CD8+ T cells may be responsible, but more work was required.

A new study[71] employed the established model of inducing peanut allergy and challenges at intervals of 4 to 10 weeks for a total of 7 challenges over a period of 36 weeks after discontinuation of FAHF-2 treatment. More than any other study I read, this one crystalizes the brilliance of the partnership between ancient medicine and contemporary science. The basic formula was developed by healers who never understood modern chemistry and biology; they just learned what worked through, I suppose, trial and error. Administering it to patients—mice in this case—is really just an extension of that tradition. The results were gratifying; the therapy showed staying power. Wonderful to me, however, is the fact that the observed results can be assayed and quantified. I love it that you can tell time by an old cathedral clock, but it's more fun when you can see the motion of the gears, pendulums, and weights that move the hands.

In this case, treated mice were protected against anaphylaxis for as long as 36 weeks compared with sham-treated mice. At that juncture, cytokine profiles of splenocytes and MLN cells and found that, even after 36 weeks, the cytokine profiles were similar to those immediately after treatment: increased IFN-γ and reduced Th2 cytokine production. As before, CD8+ T cells from FAHF-2–treated mice showed enhanced IFN-γ production, but there was no increase in the output of CD4+ cells, which, although they "are critical for proper immune cell homeostasis and host defense" can also be "troublemakers" contributing to immune and inflammatory disease.[72] This confirmed expectations that CD8+ is the dominant player and that, once more, the effect of FAHF-2 is to modulate the balance of Th1 and Th2 activity, "curing" one condition without causing another. The hope that a treatment could be administered a few times per year rather than daily or weekly would be a tremendous boon to compliance.

The study showed that a single 7-week course of FAHF-2 treatment prevented anaphylactic reactions for 6 months after therapy, 25% of a mouse's life span, a period that included 6 peanut challenges.

Approximately 9 months after therapy, only 37% of mice showed moderate reactions, whereas all sham-treated mice had severe anaphylaxis symptoms. Serum peanut-specific IgE levels were low throughout the 9-month period, in contrast to anti-IgE treatment, in which free-IgE increased 2 weeks after treatment was discontinued. Blocking antibody IgG2a levels also remained high after FAHF-2 treatment, thus interfering with mast-cell degranulation by taking up receptor space in a region on the mast cells that in allergic patients is normally dominated by a "high-affinity receptor" known as FceRI.

Thus, in addition to sustained reduction of peanut-specific IgE, increased peanut-specific IgG2a may contribute to the long-term benefits of FAHF-2 treatment by intercepting antigens before they have a chance to do any harm. These results also suggest that FAHF-2 does not induce overall immune suppression but lasting rebalancing of the ratio of IgG[ood] and igE[vil].

Both *in vivo* and *in vitro* experiments had produced evidence that the herbal formula can produce complete, long-lasting protection against peanut-induced anaphylaxis. The possibility that prolonged protection can be attained without continuous drug treatment represents a significant potential therapeutic advantage over any more conventional or unconventional therapy now envisioned.

9

Human Trials

Contemplating a Human Trial

This research didn't unfold in a straight line. By 2005, though years of research with mice lay ahead, it seemed feasible to the team that FAHF-2 would be proven safe and effective not only for mice but for people, too. The ingredients had been validated by thousands of years of medicinal use. The formula was now adjusted to avoid running afoul of FDA safety standards. Moreover, the effectiveness of the formulas in treating parasites and allergic conditions also pointed toward success.

The time had come, however, to envision how to formulate the medicines and administer them to people, and in this regard, some of the biggest hurdles weren't regulatory or scientific but cultural.

Chinese herbal preparations are typically boiled and drunk, or boiled, mashed, and combined into pills. The fact that the typical patient in this case would be a child presented an additional challenge. In pill form, WMW is taken for parasites in a regimen of 10 pills 3 times a day before meals; however, this duration is dictated by the lifecycle of the worms, not the years it might take to retrain the immune system for food allergies. For this purpose, it was calculated that 50 pills a day would be required over many months, a dreary prospect for the medical team, so they decided to first try it in liquid form. Yuck! Bitter!

This presented a problem, because substances such as triterpenes in *Ling Zhi* that make them bitter are also the active medicinal components. Dr. Li says that if her colleagues had grown up in China, where large quantities of herbs were drunk from early childhood, they would have had no problem tolerating quantities of bitter tea, but the herbal decoction was unpalatable for Western tastes. Adding sugar only made the bitterness worse. Regardless, home brewing is just a practical impossibility. A one-day therapeutic dose would take approximately 4 ounces of herbs (see chapter 3) with water enough to boil for several hours, and the BTUs it would take to boil them for that long. Multiply that daily regime by 3 to 5 years.

So, pills it was.

First Do No Harm

Testing FAHF-2 in human beings has to proceed more judiciously than in the mouse studies. Before testing for FAHF-2's protective effects, the team had to meet the first criterion of any medical therapy—to not make the patient sick in the course of treatment. Mice are rodents. People are people.

The mouse studies had established that FAHF-2 completely blocks peanut-induced anaphylaxis in mice, that mice are protected against anaphylaxis for at least 6 months, and that the effect is associated with sustained suppression of the mechanisms of allergy responses and increased levels of protection. Furthermore, there was a large margin of safety; mice fed 24 times the effective daily dose showed no signs of acute toxic effects, evidence of abnormal liver and kidney functions, abnormal complete blood cell counts, or major organ disease. Human cells tested in the laboratory demonstrated a beneficial immunomodulatory effect of FAHF-2 on peripheral blood mononuclear cells (PBMCs) from children allergic to peanut and at least one other food. These results indicate that FAHF-2 was a candidate to treat a spectrum of the most serious food allergies, not just one at a time. This would make it more useful than allergen-specific OIT, which would take years of desensitizing to one food at a time.

On the basis of the preliminary observations, the team initiated the first-ever phase-1 study to evaluate a treatment for food allergy as an FDA IND botanical drug product (IND 77,468). The drug would be given for one week.[73] This study was approved by the Mount Sinai Medical Center institutional review board, and each participant provided written informed consent before enrollment.

One major challenge to the integrity of a blinded human trial is for the researchers to remain scrupulously indifferent to anything that might create bias. Dr. Li told me that her friends give her a hard time when she refers to patients in trials as subjects rather than anything more human.

Dr. Julie Wang is one of the physicians who works directly with subjects. She walks a fine line between bedside manner and scientific detachment. She has trained herself not to speculate about whether one subject or another is receiving the drugs or the placebo. It is her job to record any ailment that subjects report, "even a stubbed toe, which obviously has nothing to do with the treatment or the placebo." Wang says that the test subjects often volunteer their own speculation, which the researchers studiously ignore. "During pollen season, they might say, 'I'm feeling better than I did last year—I must be on FAHF-2,' but all I do is write down their symptoms and forget the rest of it."

Whereas the mouse trials involved only peanut allergy, the first human trial also encompassed tree nuts, fish, and shellfish because after peanut allergies, allergies to these are least likely to be outgrown. Individuals aged 12 through 45 years of age were eligible. Their history of these allergies was documented by positive skin-test results and/or food allergen-specific IgE level. Females of childbearing potential had to either be sexually inactive or using effective birth-control measures for the duration of the study.

Candidates were excluded for acute infection; history of systemic diseases; abnormal hepatic, bone marrow, or renal function; clinically significant abnormal electrocardiogram result; current uncontrolled moderate-to-severe asthma; drug or alcohol abuse; pregnancy or lactation; and participation in another research protocol within the previous 30 days.

This was a randomized, double-blinded, placebo-controlled (neither researchers nor subjects knew who was getting FAHF-2 or placebo), dose-escalation, phase-1 trial. Three doses of FAHF-2 were used: 2.2 grams (4 tablets), 3.3 grams (6 tablets), and 6.6 grams (12 tablets) 3 times a day for 7 days—a dose range based on previous experience with FAHF-2 in animal models. Four active and 2 placebo patients were treated at each level, and doses were increased after independent review of the data from the 6 patients receiving the lower dose.

Initial evaluation consisted of a thorough medical history and physical examination, vital signs, skin-prick testing and food-specific IgE testing, baseline pulmonary function, electrocardiography, urinalysis, and routine laboratory blood tests (complete blood cell count, serum chemical analyses, renal function, liver function tests, and pregnancy test for female participants).

After initial screening, patients were prescribed either FAHF-2 or placebo for 7 days. Patients continued food-allergen avoidance for the duration of the study and were asked to refrain from other herbal medication use. Investigators spoke twice with each patient by telephone during the 7-day period to reinforce medication compliance and assess potential adverse effects. Patients were instructed to complete a symptom diary. During the final visit, the medical history was reviewed again and a final physical examination was done, including spirometry, a measurement of lung function, specifically the volume and/or speed of air that can be inhaled and exhaled. This is used to assess asthma severity. Electrocardiography and laboratory testing were also done.

Before enrollment and at the end of the week-long treatment, titrated SPTs were performed with stock peanut or individual tree nut, fish, and/or shellfish extracts, as well as negative saline controls and positive controls using a histamine base. Levels of interleukins, IFN-γ, and other pertinent cytokines were measured throughout using some of the laboratory methods described in previous chapters.

A total of 23 patients with food allergy underwent initial evaluation. Of these, 2 were excluded who had no evidence of food allergy on skin-prick testing and serum specific IgE testing, and 2 had uncontrolled asthma. No clinically significant differences were found between the FAHF-2 and placebo groups at baseline.

Nineteen patients were enrolled and randomized to FAHF-2 or placebo treatments; 1 patient withdrew from the study after the second day (sixth dose) because of an allergic reaction. Eighteen patients (12 patients in the FAHF-2 group and 6 in the placebo group) successfully completed 7 days of treatment and were included in the analyses evaluating the tolerability and safety of FAHF-2.

Escalation was allowed in a group if none of the 6 experienced a toxic effect as defined by a grade-3 adverse event (AE) attributable to the medication. The standards were adapted from the World Health Organization (WHO) standards, except that they were applied more stringently. A grade-1 "mild" AE according to the WHO was regarded as a grade-3 "severe" event for purposes of this study. If 1 of 6 patients in the FAHF-2 group had experienced such a toxic effect, then 6 additional patients (again, 4 in the FAHF-2 group and 2 in the placebo group) were added to that group and the dose escalation delayed until the additional patients completed the safety evaluation. If fewer than 2 of the 12 patients in the group experienced a dose-limiting toxic effect, the next 6 were enrolled at a higher dose. If 2 of the 12 patients experienced a dose-limiting toxic effect on any specified dose, no additional patients were to be enrolled at that dose or higher dose, pending further discussions with the independent safety reviewers.

No grade-3 AEs occurred in patients treated with FAHF-2. One patient receiving the drug reported diffuse urticaria—hives—3 hours after the sixth dose (12 tablets), but no other associated symptoms. He was instructed to stop using the study medication. The rash progressively worsened, and he was seen in a local emergency department 24 hours later. Physical examination and treatment by a dermatologist indicated this was a flare-up of atopic dermatitis unrelated to the study. The patient returned for skin-prick testing with FAHF-2 one month later, which was negative, but he had a reaction to the positive control (histamine) and no reaction to the negative control (saline); therefore, this reaction was deemed unlikely to be related to the study medication.

Of the 18 participants who completed 7 days of treatment, 1 FAHF-treated patient out of 12 (8%) reported loose bowel movements once a day on days 1 through 4, which normalized thereafter, and 1 placebo-treated patient out of 6 (17%) reported a single episode of vomiting on day 4. Neither patient required treatment.

Overall, no significant differences were found in laboratory values obtained at baseline or after completing FAHF-2 treatment. Pulmonary-function tests and electrocardiogram findings before and after treatment remained substantially constant, as did allergen-specific IgE and SPT results before and after 7 days of FAHF-2 treatment. *In vitro* treatment of patients' PBMCs with FAHF-2 showed reduced IL-5 secretion and increased IFN-g and IL-10 secretion. The conclusion? FAHF-2 is safe and well tolerated in food-allergic patients.

Extended Phase-1 Study—Inhibiting Effect on Basophils[74]

The original 7-day study was encouraging for its safety and tolerability and because underlying cellular activity pointed to favorable effects on the immune system, consistent with those from the mouse trials. It was a double-blind, placebo-controlled clinical trial, the "gold standard" because neither patients nor researchers know which subjects are getting a placebo and which ones are getting the treatment. Because subjects don't know, their beliefs and expectations don't taint the results. Because the researchers don't know either, they can't inadvertently hint to patients about what to expect and what the results will be.

A second phase-1 study was designed to evaluate safety and tolerability over a longer period of time, with additional study of physiological changes without the poking, prodding, force-feeding, blood-letting, hazardous food challenges, and, of course, dissection that can be done on mice.

Unlike the first trial, however, this was an open-label study. Each participant would receive the medication. Convinced now that FAHF-2 works (i.e., is safe and influences the underlying biochemistry in a favorable direction), Dr. Li and her colleagues wanted to study its effects on a broad set of measures. Because they couldn't regularly challenge their subjects as they had the mice, however, the researchers needed to find a biomarker that could be studied in the laboratory and dosed with antigens without risking anyone's health.

They chose the basophil. Basophils comprise less than 1% of leukocytes, but, like mast cells, are critical to allergic reactions, especially the later phases because by circulating, they provide "reinforcements" to a defense that is already underway. Unlike mast cells, which are lodged in tissue, basophils can be extracted from the blood.

The basophil-activation test (BAT) requires very small quantities of blood and does not require isolation of cells. The case for using basophils as a biomarker was buttressed by another study by Jones et al[75] showing that basophil activation was significantly reduced by 4 to 6 months of OIT and that inhibition of basophils correlated with clinical protection irrespective of IgE levels. In other words, the dogs wouldn't bark or bite every time someone knocked on the front door.

Potential subjects were screened for the same criteria listed above. In the study, participants were started on FAHF-2 (3.3 g, 6 tablets) 3 times a day for 6 months. They continued to avoid their food allergens for the duration of the study and were asked to refrain from other herbal medication use. Study investigators telephoned every other week to reinforce and confirm medication compliance and to assess potential AEs, and saw subjects every 8 weeks. As before, all participants were instructed to complete a symptom diary. At each visit, the interim medical history was reviewed, and physical examination, spirometry, electrocardiography, and laboratory studies were repeated. Although this study did not include a control group of untreated subjects, as discussed, evidence from other research suggests what a control group might have produced. Jones et al. reported that merely avoiding peanut for 6 months *does not* reduce basophil-activation responses. Like most diagnosed food-allergy patients, moreover, most of the patients in the Sinai study had avoided their food allergens for several years before enrolling in the study and yet their blood showed a high baseline level of basophil activation when exposed to antigens in the test tube. *

Studies like this are critically dependent on a consistently high-quality source of test material. The FAHF-2 used came from the same high-quality batch from the acute phase-1 study. An HPLC fingerprint of FAHF-2 was generated by Dr. Yang's team with an eye to standardizing the FAHF-2 product and to monitoring consistency and shelf life. This fingerprint helped establish the consistency of FAHF-2 used during both the phase-1 trial in July 2007 and the second study a year later.

Eighteen subjects were enrolled, but 4 withdrew: 1 because of pregnancy, 2 because of the time required and high number of tablets taken daily, and 1 with transient abdominal complaints without vomiting or diarrhea.

The median age of the patients was 16 years (range 12–27 years), and 2/3 were male. No patient was allergic only to peanut, and all but 5% had other allergic diseases, including asthma, allergic rhinitis, and atopic dermatitis.

There were no changes in hematology or chemistry laboratory values, pulmonary function, or electrocardiographic findings obtained at baseline, at 2-month intervals, or after completion of 6 months of FAHF-2 treatment. Neither were there changes in SPTs at baseline or after 6 months of FAHF-2 treatment.

One patient had an AE. She had a previous history of EoE (a form of allergic inflammation caused when white blood cells called eosinophils infiltrate the esophagus, where they don't normally appear), which had been diagnosed two years before but was not believed to have active disease and was not receiving treatment when the study began. After 5 1/2 weeks

---

* There is a misconception, promulgated even by some allergists according to reports I have gotten, that strict avoidance can make the body "forget" that it is allergic. Some people do "outgrow" their allergies, for reasons not fully understood, but "forgetting" probably has nothing to do with it.

on FAHF-2 treatment, she contacted the study coordinator to report that she had what she believed to be a recurrence of her EoE. She was instructed to discontinue FAHF-2 until her gastroenterologist could evaluate her. The gastroenterologist performed an upper endoscopy, which did reveal inflammation. After treatment for her gastric problems, the participant was restarted on FAHF-2 and completed the study with no other abdominal complaints.

BATs were performed on the blood of the other 11 patients. These tests monitor basophil expression of the protein CD63 on the cell surface. They showed a significant reduction in basophil percentages after 6 months of FAHF-2 treatment when challenged in test tubes.

These results not only suggest that long-term use of FAHF-2 safe, but also provide strong evidence that FAHF-2 may be effective in treating food allergy. As always, additional studies were needed.

10

Too Many Pills

As mentioned earlier, one of the biggest obstacles to controlling chronic disease according to medical professionals of all credentials—doctors, nurses, and pharmacists alike—is getting patients to follow their prescribed treatment—so-called compliance, or adherence. This is certainly the case with asthma. Patients often don't take their inhaled medication twice a day, as instructed, or monitor their peak flows as often as they should. They are also advised to avoid the things that trigger their disease to the greatest extent possible, but can't, or don't.

Because there is no preemptive medication for food allergies, patients are stuck with avoiding their offending foods as their sole day-to-day strategy, which has frustrations of its own. When the child is an infant and toddler, parents have a big say in his or her daily activities and eating habits. By the age of three or four, most children under the care of a conscientious doctor and diligent parents can begin to take part in their own avoidance. Many children learn to read labels very young and will alert a parent when there is danger.

At these ages, one of the greatest threats is from caregivers. One study shows that 11% of anaphylaxis incidents result from parents, babysitters, grandparents, and others feeding children the food intentionally.[76] Another study at Johns Hopkins listed a number of rationales by parents for giving a child a forbidden food, among them that they didn't believe small exposures would provoke a reaction, to see if the allergy had resolved, as "do-it-yourself immunotherapy," or that they didn't believe the diagnosis. Teenagers sometimes try forbidden foods deliberately. Then, too, only 27% of patients who experience anaphylaxis are given an epinephrine auto-injector, the most effective emergency treatment.[77] Many patients and caregivers hesitate to use epinephrine because they are fearful of side effects, especially the jolt it may give to a young heart. The conventional wisdom, however, is that epinephrine represents no threat to the child's health, especially compared to the potential for tragedy from a wait-and-see approach.

If OIT proves itself as a mainstream therapy, adherence will become an issue, although it may entail a handful of peanut M&Ms rather than a couple of puffs on an inhaler. A cure would be better.

As mentioned in chapter 8, Dr. Li and her colleagues decided early on that FAHF-2 should be delivered in pill form rather than as a decoction, or tea. "Liquid works with Chinese children who are used to drinking medicinal tea from a very young age," says Dr. Li, "for the weeks it takes to treat intestinal parasites." To "reeducate" the immune system—Dr. Li's word, not mine—and cure food allergies over many months or even years is another matter.

But how many pills? Evaporating the unrefined decoction produced a daily dose of 50 pills. This was reduced to 36 for the 6-month extension of the phase-1 human trial, during which 2 of 18 participants aged 12 to 45 dropped out because of compliance issues. Part of the problem was the time commitment involved, but the number of pills was also a factor. Unless the number could be reduced, FAHF-2 would never become a useful mass treatment. Life in food-allergy families is already stressful. The prospect of standing over a child 3 times a day to make him take 12 pills for years on end is daunting.

Water extraction was the logical first step because it mixes so well with so many things. It the "universal solvent." In the right concentrations, salt, sugar, and many other things can remain dissolved in water indefinitely. Water has its limits for separating the active ingredients in FAHF-2 from unnecessary residues from the original herbs, however.

The way forward was to make a more concentrated pill. If more of the active ingredients could be contained in a pill of the same volume and weight, then fewer of them would be necessary. How were they to do this? Scientists resort to complicated schemes based on how easily different compounds dissolve in different liquids. The idea is to remove as many impurities and inert residues from the compounds you are interested in as possible. Although the new pills may be chemically identical, however, the new formulations still must be tested for effectiveness (the purification could mangle the compounds) and safety.

Water by itself couldn't remove the impurities. However, using ethanol, which is less polar than water, they were able to further extract the active ingredients in FAHF-2 cutting the daily dose by approximately 30% while retaining efficacy and safety. Reducing a daily dose of 36 pills by 30% still leaves us with a massive number of pills to be taken at each meal, however. Dr. Li's team then used a solvent that is even less polar than ethanol: butanol.

Based on the known characteristics of FAHF-2, the team hypothesized that the less-polar solvent butanol would retain even more of the active compounds. Because butanol isn't also soluble with water, it can be separated from water and the medicinal compounds that dissolve better in butanol are attracted to that layer. Picture salad dressing made of oil, vinegar, and herbs. When the oil rises to the top, the heavier vinegar sinks to the bottom and takes the herbs with it, while the oil remains clear, although in this case, the lighter butanol would rise to the top with the active ingredients while the impurities would remain in the heavier aqueous (water) layer.

Powdered FAHF-2 extract was dissolved in distilled water and dispersed with ultrasound waves for 15 minutes, in which an electrical signal is converted into a physical vibration (called sonification), helping break apart compounds or cells. The aqueous layer was extracted with butanol 4 times in all. Each time, more of the inert residue was removed and the active ingredients became more concentrated. Drying them so they could be shaped into pills presented one additional challenge. Because butanol has a high boiling point compared to water (118° C vs. 100°C), drying would take longer, which would become a problem especially after manufacturing is scaled up. Prolonged exposure to higher heat might also "overcook" the ingredients. Ethanol's boiling point, by contrast, is only 79° C, which is why when you cook with wine or brandy, you can get rid of the alcohol without losing the flavor. The solution was to add water to the butanol, which lowered the boiling point. The combined butanol extracts of concentrated active compounds were then mixed with distilled water at a 3-to-1 ratio and evaporated under reduced pressure.

Would It Work?

It remained to be seen whether the new extract would be as potent as the less-refined versions.

After inducing peanut allergy as before, mice were treated with the new medicine, dubbed B-FAHF-2, at a dose only 1/5 by volume as had been used previously, with sham-treated mice as controls.[78] Blood was collected at the time of each challenge, and body temperatures were recorded.

B-FAHF-2 produced prolonged protection against anaphylaxis despite multiple peanut challenges. By the sixth and seventh challenges, at week 40 and 50 after the first course of therapy, half the treated mice developed score-2 mild reactions to the periodic challenges with peanut allergen. Thus, even after almost a full year, the median scores of B-FAHF-2–treated mice were significantly lower than sham-treated mice.

A second course of B-FAHF-2 treatment 8 1/2 months after the first course of treatment restored complete protection against the final challenge at week 65. Mice were therefore significantly protected for approximately 12 months, half of their life span. Protection was registered by the now-familiar clinical measures as well as by observed signs of anaphylaxis. Peanut-allergic sham-treated mice had significantly lower body temperatures compared with naïve mice following each challenge. Mean temperatures of those mice that had been treated were essentially the same as in naïve mice and significantly higher than in sham-treated mice at each of 7 challenges following the first course, and at the challenge after the second course of treatment. Plasma histamine levels after the second course of treatment were also indistinguishable from those of naïve mice following the final challenge.

Treated mice had persistently lower levels of peanut-specific IgE through week 65. Conversely, peanut-specific IgG2a (IgGood)-blocking antibody levels were significantly increased following 4 weeks of B-FAHF-2 treatment and remained significantly elevated through week 65.

It appeared, therefore, that B-FAHF-2 treatment also suppressed antigen-specific Th2 cytokine secretion and increased Th1 cytokine INF-γ secretion.

When cytokines were assayed, this was borne out. Consistent with the earlier experiments, B-FAHF-2 was shown to modulate B cell activity in the right direction—up for tolerance-related cytokines, and down for allergenic ones. More studies provided direct evidence that, in vitro, B-FAHF-2 directly suppressed peanut-primed Th2 cell, B-cell and mast-cell activities, suggesting that many mechanisms underlie B-FAHF-2's clinical effects, although the precise mechanisms remain to be determined.

No Sickness, No Death

To test B-FAHF-2 for safety apart from the therapeutic effects, mice were fed 12 times the daily dose and observed for 24 hours. None died or even got sick. Moreover, in the 2 weeks following, there were no signs of altered physical appearance or activity. Blood cell counts and serum liver/kidney function test results were all within the normal range 2 weeks after feeding. Examined under a microscope, tissue samples from the heart, lung, liver, kidney, stomach, and spleen from B-FAHF-2 mice showed nothing unusual. The B-FAHF-2-fed mice were continuously observed over a 65-week period, and none showed signs of altered physical appearance or activity.

Butanol proved so effective at extracting the useful compounds from a complex herbal formula that it points the way for tolerable treatment of food allergies. B-FAHF-2 reduced the effective daily dose for peanut-allergic mice by 80% compared to the water extract (FAHF-2) while retaining excellent efficacy and safety. The therapeutic effect is long-lasting, didn't generate resistance, and acted on multiple cells involved in the allergic response.

Additional *in vitro* research showed that B-FAHF-2 directly suppressed IgE production by a human B-cell line and activation of rat basophil leukemia (RBL) cells in dosages far below those of FAHF-2. The IC50 (dose that causes 50% inhibition) of B-FAHF-2 was **7.5-fold** lower for B-FAHF-2 than for FAHF-2. No cytotoxicity (cell damage) was observed. Because B-FAHF-2 is markedly more convenient for clinical use than is FAHF-2, the team has proposed combining B-FAHF-2 and peanut OIT, with the goal of increasing safety and efficacy of that approach. Food allery is a complicated epidemic. Meeting the needs of a broad variety of patients will require a portfolio of treatments.

11

Documenting the Quest for a Cure

M any mice die as a consequence of laboratory science. So do many trees, because of the reams of paperwork, although I suppose it might be more accurate to say these days that mounds of coal must be burned to crunch all the numbers and record the data electronically.

Any IND—FAHF-2 is known as IND 77,468—must be documented in the form of an annual report, which describes the progress that has been made to date and new studies that are being planned. For someone like me, who has only a lay appreciation of the details of such research, the IND annual report provides a useful summary of the knowledge acquired in dozens of peer-reviewed papers. Step-by-step increments are drawn together and condensed.

The October 2012 annual report for the phase-2 trial recounts screening 106 patients at 3 sites, which yielded 68 subjects—a scientific term meaning people.

Again, "first do no harm" is the paramount consideration. The most important data concerns adverse effects. Adverse effects are recorded as "definitely related," "probably related," "possibly related," and "unrelated."[79]

The data point that Dr. Li is most proud of is that not a single adverse effect was deemed definitely related to the formula under study. Of the most common symptom (gastrointestinal) 81 were reported, including vomiting, diarrhea, and abdominal pain; only 8 were deemed probably related to the medication, 41 possibly related, and 32 unrelated. Of the second most common symptoms (respiratory), only one was deemed possibly related and 74 were *un*related.

Each symptom was investigated by personal physicians as well as by participating doctors. In all, 10 subjects withdrew, 4 of them because of time constraints and difficulty with compliance, and 4 more because of recurrent abdominal pain.

Another prominent item in the annual report was something that had been mentioned in the peer-reviewed studies but that, in this more concise format, loomed larger. Though the various iterations of FAHF up-regulated the production of nonallergenic Th1 cytokines and down-regulated those of Th2, they accomplished this with no cytotoxicity to the PBMCs. That is, there was no "collateral damage" to cells that might play a critical role in maintaining a strong immune system. This adds to the appeal of herbal medicines' ability to restore balance to the bodies of mice and people without damaging anything important, as opposed to, say, antibiotics, which we now know destroy good bacteria as well as harmful ones, something associated in theory with one aspect of the rise of the allergy epidemic.

Refining FAHF-2 Allows Researchers to Isolate and Understand Effectiveness of Active Compounds

Using butanol to refine FAHF-2 not only makes it possible to reduce the daily dosage from 30 pills to 6—a must for eventual clinical use—but also makes possible characterization and purification of the active compounds. This allows us to understand which of the ingredients are doing what.

The annual report documents this activity in great detail: Isolation of 4 fractional compounds from B-FAHF-2 based on their polarity using a "preparative HPLC system" showed that the different compounds contributed to inhibiting the allergic response in different ways. The "alkaloid-rich fraction 2 (F2) inhibited IgE production and mast-cell degranulation *in vitro*" while fractions 3 and 4 (F3, F4), rich in *flavonoids* and *triterpenes*, inhibited TNF-α production, which contributes to inflammation. Two compounds from F2 demonstrated that "*berberine* is the most potent active compound in F2 that inhibits IgE production, mast-cell degranulation, and Th2 cytokine production". Using HPLC to create chemical "fingerprints," the peaks of F3 and F4 were found to correspond to those of *Ling-Zhi* (*Ganoderma luciderm*), the magic mushroom. So far, 15 compounds have been isolated and characterized from *Ling Zhi* itself. We are a long way from the story of the white snake.

B-FAHF-2 was also analyzed for heavy metals, pesticides, and microbes and was found to fall within acceptable limits. In addition, the placebo tablets had to meet safety standards.

Thus, the stage was set for a new trial within precise parameters: 18 patients randomized to receive 4 tablets of B-FAHF-2 bid (twice a day) for 7 days, double-blind. Corn-flour placebo tablets are produced by the same manufacturer that produced the B-FAHF-2 active drug.

The report describes the procedure in great detail: "The initial evaluation will consist of a thorough medical history and physical examination; vital signs—blood pressure, heart and breathing rate, body temperature; prick-skin testing to peanut, individual tree nuts, sesame and/or individual fish or shellfish; total IgE level; peanut-specific, tree nut-specific, sesame-specific, and/or fish- or shellfish-specific IgE level; baseline spirometry; electrocardiogram; urinalysis; and pregnancy test and routine laboratory blood tests (complete blood count, serum chemistries, renal function, liver function tests). Subjects will be instructed to complete a symptom diary while they are participating in the trial. The clinical site investigators will be in direct telephone contact with each subject approximately every other day. Also, a study physician will be on call to discuss possible AEs by telephone. During the final visit of the acute phase-1 trial, the investigators will review the larger status of subject health, including the symptom diary. The final visit will incorporate a physical examination, vital signs, spirometry, electrocardiogram, urinalysis, and routine laboratory blood tests (complete blood count, serum chemistries, renal function, liver function tests)."

Prior to the start of the acute phase-1 trial, aliquots of peripheral blood mononuclear cells will be treated *in vitro* with B-FAHF-2 to determine the direct effect of B-FAHF-2 or its compounds on T-cell cytokine profiles and histamine release by basophils. Furthermore, B-FAHF-2 effects on cytokine and transcription factor gene expression and regulation including epigenetic regulation of T cells will be determined.

The FDA has now given approval for using B-FAHF-2 to replace FAHF-2 for the clinical study. A new acute phase-1 study will be initiated, but because FAHF-2 showed excellent safety data, the team doesn't have to go back to square one to establish safety. The dose will be 8 tablets daily to ease clinical administration and compliance and to allow a longer duration of treatment that is more comparable to the murine experiments. {Note: Documentation is being prepared as of this writing}

PART THREE

The Future

As we await the results of the latest phase of FAHF-2 trials, it's not too early to peer into the future and think about other dimensions suggested by Dr. Li's work. Each of the final five chapters focuses on a different element of the ongoing story, from very practical extensions of the research just described to breathtaking concepts suggested by new insights into the nature of the immune system.

12. Multiple Food Allergies for the Price of One

OIT may prove practical for a certain proportion of food-allergic patients—probably those who are allergic to a single allergen and have no problems with eosinophils in their digestive tracts—but what of those who have many food allergies? Quite apart from the difficulties of assessing the progress for any individual allergen, there's the problem of continually subjecting these patients to known irritants. The alternative is to modulate the immune system itself.

13. From One Generation to the Next

Many parents wonder how life-threatening allergies can emerge mysteriously in very small children. Although a genetic predisposition to allergies is accepted science, the new science of epigenetics is starting to reveal how the environment, diet, and behavior can affect the way our genes are expressed and that these subtle alterations can be passed to offspring. This chapter not only documents how detrimental changes can be passed on but also shows that it may be possible to reverse such transmission in the future.

81

14. Beyond Food Allergies

One of the most exciting things about the East-meets-West paradigm is that we not only can see that these herbal compounds work but can also determine why they work. Instead of measuring the effect of a single molecule on a single molecule or a single pathway, we can see how a complex compound works on multiple compounds and pathways that are part of other pathologies. This chapter looks at the way Dr. Li's research is finding currency outside the strict realm of allergies.

15. Treating Severe Allergic Diseases: Three Cases from Private Clinical Practice

As Dr. Scott Sicherer tells his colleagues, in China, TCM is just medicine. In her private clinic, Dr. Li regularly uses medicines that are approved as supplements to treat severe allergic diseases apparently with great success. This chapter gives anecdotal accounts of three successful treatments of debilitating and life-threatening allergic cases that have restored joy to the lives of young patients.

16. The Slow Road to Clinical Practice

This final chapter grapples with the shortcomings of traditional allergy treatment and research and outlines a possible roadmap for accelerating the practice of integrative medicine—the adoption of TCM-based drugs by a wider population of traditional allergists.

12

Multiple Food Allergies for the Price of One

Although peanut allergy gets most of the attention, there remain seven other *major* food allergens—dairy, tree nuts, eggs, shellfish, fish, soy, wheat—and dozens more minor ones. Any of these has the capacity to provoke anaphylaxis—that is, a combination of symptoms in more than one organ system (skin, respiratory, digestive), which can be life-threatening. Most research into desensitization against food allergies has concentrated on one allergen at a time. Unlike immunotherapy for environmental allergies, for which multiple allergens can be injected together, experiments with OIT for food allergies have concentrated on single allergens because of the different profiles of the different foods. Approximately 20% of children outgrow their peanut, shellfish, fish, and tree-nut allergies, whereas 80% outgrow their milk and egg allergies.[80] Studies are inconclusive for milk allergies in particular as to whether OIT is responsible for desensitization or whether it has taken place on its own since 80% outgrow them.[81]

Then, too, the proteins in different foods may be altered by cooking, sometimes making them less allergenic, or sometimes more. Ara h2, which is one of the big-three peanut allergens, seems to be strengthened by roasting (the dominant method of preparation in the United States) and weakened by boiling, frying, and pickling, which are more common in Korea. Ara h1 and Ara h3, however, are not affected, so this doesn't constitute much protection.[82] The important variable between these components and the less-allergenic Ara h6 and Ara h8 is that the more dangerous proteins are harder to digest and are more likely to survive intact and be absorbed, allowing them to circulate and cause systemic reaction. For kids with peanut allergies, no method of cooking changes the proteins sufficiently, but baking eggs or milk may help the child allergic to these foods.

Between the different molecular profiles of various allergens, the tendency for patients to outgrow at different rates, and so on, assembling a homogeneous sample for a single food study is hard enough. For multiple allergens, it would be far more difficult.

One answer is to attack the problem from the other direction—the production of antibodies without regard for specific allergies. All these allergies have something in common: the Th2-IgE mediated response. The most promising line of OIT for multiple food allergies uses omalizumab to speed the process of desensitization. This research is being conducted under the direction of Dr. Kari Nadeau of Stanford.

Omalizumab works by binding a particular epitope on the handle-like portion of IgE antibodies so they can no longer attach to their allergen-specific high-affinity receptors on the mast cell. They become, in effect, square pegs that can no longer fit in their round holes. This gives IgG(ood)4 blocking antibodies the chance to occupy these receptors without competition from IgE(vil). Because all IgE antibodies have the same handle, it should work with all of them. Thus, the doctor can theoretically supply all the allergens at once, and all the IgE will be rendered harmless long enough for the IgG4 blocking antibodies to occupy all the receptors. This universal effect has led to omalizumab being studied for off-label treatment of other allergic conditions besides asthma, particularly chronic urticaria—really bad recurring hives.

Promising though this combination therapy sounds, omalizumab has a few drawbacks, as mentioned earlier. One is that it is itself a protein to which a few people can become allergic. Another is cost, approximately $1000 per month, possibly forever, which makes it economical to use mainly for severe asthmatics who would otherwise be hospitalized frequently, costing their insurance companies much more. A third drawback is that omalizumab may not improve on the likely weakness of OIT in general—namely, that it only wears out current Th2 cells but its effects may be temporary. Although OIT does inhibit basophil activity for a period,[83] which helps reduce reactivity, the major food allergies often last a lifetime, even without any exposure. Once desensitization is achieved, it may be possible to maintain it with doses of the offending food only, not the $1000 drug. Annoying though it may be to take daily doses of single foods to maintain desensitization, having to incorporate peanuts, egg, wheat, and shrimp into one's everyday diet, to name just one combination, will require considerable culinary ingenuity, however.

A newer foray into combination therapy is the brainchild of Dr. Nadeau and Dr. Li, using FAHF-2 as the adjunct in the place of omalizumab. I had the privilege of sitting at lunch with the two of them and watching them outline the study on the back of a napkin.[84] It must be said that the science of food allergies is too new and patient phenotypes are too varied to concentrate all the funding and scientific talent too early in the process. It is very likely that food-allergy patients will be varied enough so that treatment will entail a range of methods. {Note: another therapy called Viaskin®, or the "peanut patch", in which measured doses of peanut extract are applied to the skin, is in trials at various medical centers, including Mount Sinai.}

The sole trial of a single therapy for multiple food allergies is being conducted by Dr. Li and colleagues at Mount Sinai and in Dallas at the University of Texas Southwestern Medical Center and Children's Medical Center. They began a new subproject of their phase-1 trial[85] to test butanol-refined FAHF-2 with subjects aged 6 to 45 who are allergic to one or more foods including peanut, tree nut, sesame, fish, or shellfish as documented by a positive skin test and/or food allergen-specific IgE level for the allergens. [The protocol for the experiment reads: "The initial evaluation will consist of a thorough medical history and physical examination; vital signs; prick skin testing to peanut, individual tree nuts, sesame, and/or individual fish or shellfish; total IgE level; peanut-specific, tree nut-specific, sesame-specific, and/or fish- or shellfish-specific IgE level; baseline spirometry; electrocardiogram; urinalysis; pregnancy test and routine laboratory blood tests (complete blood count, serum chemistries, renal function, liver function tests)."] Individuals with a history of anaphylaxis to these allergens were excluded (the object of the trial being not to cure the subjects but to examine the underlying functioning of the immune system) along with many other immune disorders and other medical conditions. Subjects will keep symptom diaries in addition to being in regular touch with study personnel.

Opening up this test to a spectrum of allergies also makes it easier to recruit subjects who meet the desired parameters. This is, in a way, the inverse of the murine model of testing. With mice, it made sense to induce allergies to a lone allergen, instead of several, and to treat them with single drug.

If this test succeeds, it will assess several things. First, it will further establish the safety of B-FAHF-2. Second, it will show that the up-regulation of Th1 cytokines and production of IgG antibodies and inhibition of Th2-IgE was general, not specific to peanuts.

13

From One Generation to the Next

"What did I do wrong?"

Many mothers of food-allergic children ask themselves that question continually from the time of diagnosis. Although the tendency of allergies to run in families is long established, the onset of life-threatening food allergies in a new generation is a shock even in families with a history of environmental allergies and asthma. Food allergies become the basis of a blame game. Mothers, fathers, in-laws—no one's genes or neurotic tendencies escape scrutiny. Privately, however, (or in the extended privacy of closed Facebook groups where I meet them), mothers pick over their gestational diets, medications they took or allowed to be given to their children, whether or not they breast-fed, how long they breast-fed; these and many other things must have been their own fault, they believe.

Self-recrimination, however, is not only a recipe for personal misery but is also wide of the mark. There is likely no single maternal behavior that has a one-to-one relationship to a child's allergies. The conventional wisdom on maternal diet—to eat certain foods, especially peanuts, or avoid them—has flip-flopped, and continuing research is equivocal. Other factors such as caesarian delivery and use of antibiotics indicate that with disruption of the natural microbe environment in a newborn, the immune system is disturbed along with it, but until now, who was to know? And let's give the moms a break. What choice did they have? These were mostly life-saving interventions, although many caesarians have been performed for "convenience." Attempts to restore a measure of balance through supplements such as probiotics and vitamins are not yet at the point where there is any clear road to correction.

Allergies do appear to get worse in succeeding generations: sneezing leads to wheezing, which leads to anaphylaxis. As mentioned in chapter 1, Dr. Susan Prescott has written that the allergy epidemic is likely the product of multiple assaults on our skin, sinuses, lungs, and digestive systems—anywhere our immune systems confront the environment. Furthermore, these assaults may accumulate from one generation to the next as toxins affect gene expression—not the genes themselves—a process called epigenetics, or "above the genome." Chris Faulk, a postdoctoral fellow studying environmental epigenetics and evolution, writes in an online article: "We know that environmental changes by toxicant exposure, stress, nutrition, and other factors can alter the epigenetic marks of many body tissues, including the gametes, and so an intergenerational epigenetic effect can be seen."[86] Thus, a child's asthma may be attributable in part to the mother's life in a city with high levels of "black carbon" from diesel fumes[87] or to a grandmother's smoking habit.[88] Families with no recorded history of allergies may become allergic, and mild allergies can get worse. My own surmise is that if humans can share 99% of our genome with mice, we can also share genetic tendencies with other human beings and that a family history with no known tendency to allergies is just a few gene expressions away from one that does have allergies. This is not the same as Lamarckism, named for Jean-Baptiste Lamarck, "who, beginning in the early 1800 s [sic], put forth the hypothesis that giraffes could pass on long necks to their offspring by stretching their own necks throughout their lives…"[89] It is instead the subtle influence of chemicals on the biochemical processes that comprise the immune system.

The bright side of Prescott's thesis is that the epigenetic cascade that has caused an epidemic of allergies and other noncommunicable inflammatory diseases didn't really start all that long ago and so might be at least partially correctible over a relatively brief time frame as well.

Toward Intergenerational Correction

The possibility of curing food allergies and passing the change on to the next generation was demonstrated in a 2009 study by Dr. Li and her Mount Sinai colleagues.[90] After peanut allergy was induced in female mice by the now-familiar method, they were bred with naïve males. A subset of these mothers received low doses of peanut and adjuvant cholera toxin during pregnancy and lactation.

At the age of 5 weeks, the offspring were challenged intragastrically with peanut extract delivered directly through a tube. This was the first exposure to the peanut allergens, so any reaction at all would indicate that allergy can be inherited, but any difference in the degree of reaction would also indicate that protection could also be inherited.

The results were dramatic: 80% of those offspring whose mothers had not received the low doses of peanuts experienced anaphylaxis, compared to just 24% of those that had. There were corresponding changes in body temperature—lower in the more allergic mice, closer to normal in the less reactive. Concentrations of the "good" blocking antibody IgG2 were greater in the offspring of the mothers that had been dosed with the peanut-adjuvant dosing. Production of Th2 cytokines associated with peanut allergies was significantly lower in the offspring of treated mothers than in those of naïve mothers. This suggested that the right intervention might also mitigate the transmission of the allergy in humans, although it would be impractical to do the same experiment in prospective mothers.

Was this change the result of what we might call "corrective epigenetics," or could some other phenomenon have been at work, such as milk from lactating mothers? Dr. Li says, "This is an excellent question. We have not fed pups on sham mothers yet, but we looked at the neonatal spleen DNA methyltion status and found hyper-methylation (repression) of IL-4 promotion at CpG sites* of pups from mothers fed peanuts and cholera toxin, even before peanut sensitization." A paper recounting this study is being prepared as of this writing.

A 2010 experiment[91] using the herbal asthma drug ASHMI—also developed by Dr. Li and her team—lent additional credence to the idea that the heritability of allergies can be blocked by intervention. ASHMI is an extract of 3 herbs—*Ling-Zhi, Ku-Shen (Radix Sophora flavescentis)*, and *Gan-Cao (Radix Glycyrrhiza uralensis)*—that exhibits a "broad spectrum of therapeutic effects on the major pathogenic mechanisms of asthma—airway hyperreactivity, pulmonary inflammation, and airway remodeling—as well as downregulating TH2 responses and direct modulation of airway smooth muscle contraction."

---

*CpG sites are regions of DNA where a cytosine nucleotide occurs next to a guanine nucleotide. This is part of the epigenome, the "clothing" of the DNA, described in chapter 1, whose response to certain stimuli determines gene expression—that is, turns the gene on or off.

To induce asthma, researchers sensitized female mice intraperitoneally—injection into the peritoneal cavity—twice with ovalbumin (OVA) and alum followed by 3 weekly intratracheal challenges with OVA. Allergic airway responses were studied. The now-asthmatic females were treated with ASHMI for 6 weeks, and controls were left untreated. Naïve females constituted an additional control group. The females were then mated with naïve males. Twelve-day-old offspring from each group received 3 consecutive daily intranasal OVA challenges. Two days later, offspring were sacrificed and bronchoalveolar lavage (BAL)* and lung histology were performed. Serum OVA antibodies and cytokine profiles were also assessed. Following the third challenge, total numbers of BAL macrophages, eosinophils, lymphocytes, and neutrophils in the asthmatic but untreated offspring were significantly higher than in BAL of offspring of naïve mothers. The offspring of untreated asthmatic mothers also contained many airway mucus cells. In contrast, the BAL cells from offspring of mothers who had received ASHMI treatment were essentially the same as those of their mothers, no mucus cells were present, and the cytokine profiles were essentially healthy. ASHMI also "significantly suppressed Th2 cytokine production by human PBMCs from patients with asthma."[92]

A 2011 study[93] presents explicit suggestion of the epigenetic effects of ASHMI. A group of OVA-allergic-asthmatic female mice were treated with either ASHMI, dexamethasone (a corticosteroid widely used to control asthma), or water (sham) for 7 weeks. Genomic DNA isolated from lung tissues, collected immediately and 8 weeks post therapy, was bisulfite converted and amplified using polymer-chain-reaction (PCR) technology to study methylation within IFN-γ and IL-4 promoters through pyrosequencing.

Immediately following therapy, methylation at the IFN- promoter was significantly decreased in ASHMI group as compared to sham groups, and to the steroid-group lung tissues, whereas methylation in the IL-4 promoter was significantly increased when compared to the steroid group. The decreases in methylation persisted for at least 8 weeks post therapy. Methylation of CpG at the IL-4 promoter in the lungs of the ASHMI group was significantly higher than in the steroid group. They conclude: "ASHMI resets epigenetic modulation of *IFN-γ* and *IL-4* expression which is favorable for long-term tolerance induction."

---

*A bronchoscope is passed into the lungs. Fluid is squirted into the lungs and then collected for study.

A subsequent experiment[94] examining food allergy instead of allergic asthma used B-FAHF-2 as the protective agent with the additional element of determining whether there might also be some benefit with egg allergy, as 70% of peanut-sensitive infants are also sensitive to egg. As before, female mice were sensitized with peanut, then treated with B-FAHF-2 or sham and mated with naïve males. At 5 weeks, offspring were sensitized with egg white and cholera toxin epicutaneously (injections into the skin) 3 times, a week apart. Offspring of mothers that received sham treatment before conception showed significantly higher egg-specific IgE levels than those of naïve mothers. The offspring of B-FAHF-2–treated mothers showed significant suppression of egg-specific IgE compared to the offspring of sham-treated mothers and were essentially the same as naïve offspring.

These results suggest that in addition to its potential as a therapeutic botanical drug, B-FAHF-2 may also have potential for treating food-allergic women prior to conception.

Unfortunately, further investigations of this kind are limited by bias against novelty both for funding and publication. Funding for basic research is generally directed at cures, not prevention. Journals prefer to publish research conducted in discrete steps rather than big leaps, even when those leaps can be convincingly engineered into the scope of an experiment.

Predicting Transmission of Food Allergies

Although maternal allergies are considered a risk factor for food allergies in the next generation, the mechanism is unknown; however, new mouse research by Ying Song et al,[95] points to the chance that heritability of food allergies can be predicted. Five-week-old offspring of peanut-allergic mothers were sensitized with peanut and cholera toxin for 4 weeks, then challenged with peanut. Sensitized offspring of naïve mothers served as a control. They were assessed for anaphylactic reactions, peanut-specific IgE in their blood, and splenocyte and mesenteric MLN cell production of IFN-γ, IL-4, IL-5, IL-10, and IL-17. In addition, the extent of gene expression—CpG methylation—of the IL-4 promoter gene in the offspring's MLN cells was measured. Methylation is a mechanism to regulate how specific genes in the DNA helix do different things at different times (gene expression), as mentioned in the first chapter.

Offspring of the peanut-allergic mothers exhibited significantly higher IgE levels at week 4, as well as more symptoms and lower core body temperature post challenge compared to offspring of normal mothers. Their lymph cells produced significantly more Th2 cytokines and fewer Th1 cytokines than cells from offspring of normal mothers. Reduced methylation at IL-4 promoter was also found. Dr. Song told me that high methylization at a couple of specific sites on the IL-4 gene has now been linked with 90% certainty of allergenicity in offspring. If there were a safe way to treat these mothers who are likely to transmit food allergy epigenetics to their children, it might be possible to reverse the transmission of allergies.

Replicating in women the process of low-dosing mice with adjuvant cholera toxin is fraught with ethical and practical obstacles, to say the least, but what if a derivative of cholera toxin could be employed that retained the binding abilities of the full toxin without the toxic effects?

As it happens, there is such a thing. A subunit of cholera toxin called cholera toxin-B (CTB) is the component that first binds to the mucosa. It is considered "an efficient mucosal carrier molecule for the generation of immune responses to linked antigens," with the added benefit that it possesses immunosuppressing qualities of its own.[96] Other researchers learned this the hard way when they tried to induce peanut allergies in mice using CTB instead of cholera toxin and it didn't work. Dr. Li says, "This gave us a clue that CTB might induce tolerance."

One of the studies was "Peanut Tolerance in Offspring of Female Mice Fed Peanut and Cholera Toxin B Subunit Is Associated with Epigenetic Regulation of Foxp3 Promoter and Induction of Mucosal Foxp3 and IL-10 Gene Expression" by Yiqun Hui, Ying Song, and others from Mount Sinai, which was presented at the AAAAI meetings in February of 2013. Dr. Kari Nadeau of Stanford calls Foxp3 genes "peacekeeping" cells and says that children lacking them have more severe allergies, asthma, gastrointestinal diseases, and type-1 diabetes than children with lower levels.[97] IL-10 is an important immunoregulator in the digestive tract and inhibits synthesis of certain inflammatory cytokines.[98]

Having previously reported that maternal consumption of peanut plus nontoxic CTB during pregnancy and subsequent lactation induced tolerance to peanut in mouse offspring, they investigated the potential association of epigenetic changes for inducing tolerance.

Peanut-allergic female mice were either fed low doses of peanut plus CTB or sham-treated during pregnancy and lactation. Intestines were collected from these and naïve offspring. Through a process called quantitative PCR, FoxP3 and IL-10 gene expression were analyzed. DNA methylation of the FoxP3 promoter region was analyzed by bisulfite sequencing PCR. Data were analyzed using one-way ANOVA followed by Bonferroni's tests (statistical methods for excluding random results).

Levels of intestinal IL-10 gene expression were significantly higher in peanut-tolerant offspring than in the allergic and naïve offspring. Intestinal Foxp3 expression in the peanut-tolerant offspring also rose compared to naïve and peanut-allergic ones, respectively. Analysis of DNA methylation revealed decreased methylation levels at the CpG250 FoxP3 promoter site in intestines from the tolerant offspring compared to allergic and naïve offspring. No differences were detected at the other 4 CpG sites.

The team concluded that CTB as an adjuvant for peanut immunotherapy appears to be effective and safe in generating oral tolerance in the offspring of sensitized mice.

Given the safety of CTB and the success of inducing tolerance in new generations of mice, this approach holds the prospect of a sea change in the allergy epidemic. Dr. Li says, "Ying's data support our hypothesis. If we can desensitize the allergic mother safely, we may be able to provide trans-generational benefits. We believe this is important because it may be able to reverse the peanut-allergy epidemic."

If this research pans out, fewer mothers will ask the question, "What did I do wrong?"

14

Beyond Food Allergies

One of the more tantalizing aspects of Dr. Li's work is its potential for treating conditions beyond allergies. Though allergies have proliferated in populations around the world, for people who don't have them or whose allergies can be minimized with relatively inexpensive measures, allergies don't sound like public enemy number one. Disordered immunity has now been linked to a much wider set of noncommunicable diseases (NCDs) that raise more eyebrows, and indeed more money, than allergies, however. Allergies may function as a kind of early warning system for NCDs, like a canary in a coal mine. Dr. Susan Prescott says, "[A]s the most common and earliest-onset NCD, the epidemic of allergic diseases points to specific vulnerability of the developing immune system to modern environmental change. Indeed, many environmental risk factors implicated in the rise of other NCDs have been shown to mediate their effects through immune pathways." Put another way, if environmental changes are doing this much damage to people who have allergies, isn't it reasonable to suppose that they might be hurting the nonallergic in other ways?

Dr. Prescott writes, "The innate immune system provides a clear example of this convergence, with evidence that physical activity, nutrition, pollutants, and the microbiome all influence systemic inflammation through Toll-like receptor pathways (notably Toll-like receptor 4), with downstream effects on the risk of insulin resistance, obesity, cardiovascular risk, immune diseases, and even mood and behavior."[99]

Dr. Renata Engler is also intrigued by this thesis. She commented in notes to me after reviewing the manuscript of this book:

The growing evidence that chronic inflammation is a key player in the major killer diseases is I believe a major 21st century medicine paradigm shift. The hypothesis that allergic individuals may have an increased risk for cardiovascular disease has yet to be tested but is a strong candidate. Chronic sinusitis and periodontal disease increase risk of cardiovascular disease; there is considerable evidence in the literature for this. Integrative medicine approaches to cardiovascular disease prevention include careful attention to dental health, underlying sources of chronic infection and inflammation. The non-specific marker of inflammation known as C-reactive protein (CRP) is a biomarker of cardiovascular inflammation risk with hyperlipidemia. Better drugs are needed to downregulate inflammation without undermining appropriate immune defenses. What if the TCM therapies that have shown such potential in modulating the immune system for treating allergies could also be applied to other conditions?

In a book called *The Genius Within: Discovering the Intelligence of Every Living Thing*, author Frank T. Vertosick Jr. (Harcourt, New York 2002) wrote, "The immune system must learn and recall billions, perhaps trillions, of different molecular patterns. Our lives depend on its ability to make instant discriminations between friend and foe, not an easy task." That capability is a wondrous thing, but when it goes wrong, it is also terrifying. The huge cast of T cells, B cells, mast cells, basophils, and the cytokines that regulate their behavior are like a stock company in a series of dramas. In a person with intestinal parasites, IgE wears a white hat and plays the hero. In a food allergy patient, it wears a black hat and plays the villain. We need treatments that can modulate excesses and insufficiencies without creating new problems. To paraphrase Dr. Li, we want to make bad boys into good boys without turning good girls bad.

The growing database of herbs that Dr. Li is compiling at Mount Sinai provides an intriguing foundation for new generations of potential treatments for a broad range of diseases. In making the leap from intestinal parasites to food allergies, Dr. Li found a treatment that seems to work, but in exploring the underlying biochemistry, trying to find out why it works, she found clues to possible shortcuts for treatment of diseases that are non-allergic but that also entail malfunctions of the immune system.

Several projects now underway at Sinai demonstrate the possibilities for treating debilitating diseases without the destructive side effects that accompany conventional immune suppression.

I am reporting these experiments not because they represent the prospect of any immediate breakthroughs across a broad spectrum of diseases. Exciting though the experiments are, the odds are against success. My great friend Dr. Mark Cullen of Stanford, who read this manuscript, got hung up on this point:

> I am always a little leery of the wistful "look how far this could go" speculation, which has become taboo in scientific writing. Since every single biologic process is tied to a trillion others, speculation about how control of one pathway might positively influence others is tempting, but it almost never pans out when challenged. The sections on Crohn's and cancer are too great a leap—I doubt Dr. Li will make contributions to those fields, sorry, and may tempt readers to draw the wrong conclusions. Asthma looks far more likely to bear fruit, but you'd be amazed how wrong most such speculations have proved to be historically. Ask any friend in pharma R&D!

Thank you, Dr. Cullen. And I wouldn't be amazed.

With Mark's admonition in mind, I'd like to point out that whatever happens may well yield greater insight into the physiological mechanisms at work. Dr. Sicherer at Mount Sinai said that Dr. Li's research has already taught us things about the immune system.

The Western pharmacopeia is full of botanical derivatives that do work, which is one of the reasons that biodiversity is so critical. Who knows what matches remain to be made between in the molecules of herbs and flowers on one continent and the T cells of sick individuals on another? The classical physicians of China did a lot of research and development for us. They showed us that certain botanicals work for certain things. Contemporary scientists can show us how those botanicals work, and by doing so, they give us clues to still other applications.

Inflammatory Bowel Disease

Among the doctors who are now collaborating with Dr. Li is David Dunkin, a gastroenterologist at Mount Sinai who spends four days a week doing research and one day mainly treating young patients with Crohn's disease and ulcerative colitis, which fall under the umbrella of inflammatory bowel disease. They have similar symptoms to one another—abdominal pain, rectal bleeding, diarrhea, weight loss, fever, and skin and eye involvement—but they differ in the way they affect different parts of the intestinal tract.[100]

Crohn's has been a focal point of research at Sinai for many decades and is named for gastroenterologist Dr. Burrill Bernard Crohn, who worked there. In 1932, working with two other colleagues, Crohn described a series of patients with inflammation of the terminal ileum, the area most commonly affected by the illness.[101] Dunkin says that he can diagnose Crohn's children very quickly because they are characteristically very pale, thin, and below average in growth. Failure to thrive is common.

Crohn's is considered an autoimmune disease. The roster of cytokines with which you are now familiar from earlier chapters may be directed at any tissue between the esophagus and the rectum, resulting in chronic destructive inflammation. As with food allergies, there is no cure, although Crohn's and colitis can be held in check by blocking the production of cytokines and suppressing inflammation with steroids. The trouble with these remedies, however, is that, as is the case with allergies, they are very blunt instruments. Systemic steroids block good cytokines along with bad and can have a debilitating effect on defenses against infections.

For children with active disease, life isn't much fun. "They have to stay home or in the hospital and typically take these strong medicines three times a day," says Dunkin. "And with chronic symptoms like diarrhea, they don't much feel like being around other kids."

Dunkin's research took a new direction when Dr. Li called him and pointed out that her research showed that FAHF-2 inhibited production of TNF-α, which was discussed in chapters 6 and 11. Dr. Li knew that high levels of TNF-α were also associated with Crohn's. According to Bellanti et al., TNF-α increases the transport of white blood cells to inflamed sites and activates neutrophils and eosinophils.[102] This induces tissue-degrading enzymes, the results of which are visible to anyone who sees endoscopic photographs of ulcers of the affected tissue. They look to me like what would happen to your skin if you rubbed it with sandpaper.

Dr. Li and Dr. Dunkin discussed whether it was possible to modulate the immune system for Crohn's as had been case with food allergies. He took blood and gut tissue samples from new patients who had been diagnosed but not yet treated, and he examined the samples for the cytokines they produced. When FAHF-2 was added to these tissues, the inflammatory cytokines were reduced.

In vitro research has since confirmed the modulating effects of FAHF-2 for Crohn's patients as well as allergic ones, and a mouse study has also had encouraging results. Dunkin says that his research has excited patients. "They ask how the Chinese study is going, but I have to caution them it will be years before there's any realistic prospect of treatment."

Note: A clinical study described as follows, is now underway at Mount Sinai:

> The purpose of this study is to see if inflammatory cytokines (markers or chemicals in the blood/tissue that are associated with active inflammatory bowel disease) will be affected by the addition of Chinese herbal medicines that are added to cultures of blood cells or tissue specimens from the colon. A blood sample will be drawn at the time of endoscopy. The blood sample will be used to obtain serum and white blood cells. The colonic (taken from the large intestine/colon) sample will be used to obtain tissue cells.[103]

Organ Rejection

One immune disorder that has spawned research under Dr. Li's auspices is very different from any other. Unlike allergies, in which the immune system turns against otherwise innocuous proteins in the environment and diet, or autoimmune diseases, in which the body attacks itself, in this case, the antigen is deliberately introduced for the purposes of saving lives. This represents the supreme contest between modern technical medical capabilities and the best the immune system has to offer—organ transplantation. Without concerted efforts to suppress its action, the immune system regards the new tissue as a massive virus, microbe, or allergen, and sets out to destroy it.

Surgeons have dreamed of transplanting organs and limbs for centuries, but except for corneas, the first successful organ transplant was only done in 1954, a kidney from one identical twin to the other. Because the twins' genes were the same, organ rejection was not an issue.

Transplantation between non-twins would have to wait for the development of immune suppressants that were safe and effective enough to be used daily for a lifetime. Cortisone has too many side effects. It was not until 1970, when cyclosporine was discovered in the fungus *Tolypodadium inflatum*, that surgeons acquired a medication suitable to make transplantation the relatively commonplace procedure it has become. Another drug, sirolimus/rapamycin was first found in the bacterium *Streptomyces hygroscopicus* on Easter Island.[104]

Although better post-transplantation clinical care and a larger repertoire of immunosuppression approaches have reduced short-term illness and lowered rates of acute organ rejection, these remain a persistent threat. Moreover, immunosuppressant drugs can cause a range of toxic side effects.[105]

Adapting an ancient herbal preparation to procedures that have been tenable for only 40 years may seem unlikely, but Dr. Jessica Reid-Adam has been exploring this possibility for several years in collaboration with Dr. Peter Heeger, her mentor at Mount Sinai and a transplant immunologist, and Dr. Li.

Dr. Reid-Adam is a pediatric nephrologist. That is, she specializes in kidney disease in children and spends much of her time treating end-stage renal failure. Her typical patient, or patient's parents, face just three choices—dying, dialysis, or transplant. Of these, transplantation is the best, in her estimation. "Dialysis means spending hours being hooked up to a machine at a dialysis center three times a week. There is home dialysis, but it requires a certain amount of room and a good deal of discipline."

When Jessica began her nephrology fellowship after completing training in pediatrics, she didn't have a research agenda. Her ambition was to work with patients, but research was a necessary part of her training. Her fellowship director, Dr. Jeff Saland, had heard Xiu-Min Li give a talk and suggested that Jessica get in touch with Dr. Li to see if there was something in TCM that might be applied in organ transplantation.

98

"Xiu-Min said she had a database of herbs and that I should see which ones sounded like they might apply to the kidneys," says Reid-Adam.

Transplantation presents a number of terrible challenges, apart from acquiring compatible organs. "Some of our patients are transplanted under the age of two."

Patients must be closely monitored for any signs of rejection and must take large amounts of immune-suppressing drugs. Moreover, the life expectancy of an individual organ is limited—typically to 5–10 years, although one patient known to Dr. Reid-Adam still has a kidney with no signs of failure after 18 years. "Most of them get an adult organ," she says. "This is not a problem surgically—all the veins and arteries connect. The real difficulty is the immune suppression. An allergy is a reaction to proteins that can be measured in micrograms. A kidney is usually 125 grams or more—5 ounces of foreign tissue in a child weighing 20 pounds."

The drugs present an additional problem: "The immune systems of small children are immature. At least an adult has some degree of protection against infection even after their immunity is suppressed. Children don't have time to develop this capacity, which makes them even more vulnerable to incidental infection and certain types of cancer."

Also, current immunosuppressants have little or no effect on memory T cells formed to react to the donated tissue, which is problematic because the transplanted organ is always there. The immune response will never go away. As Dr. Reid-Adam and her coauthors say in their first major publication, "Taken together, these observations support the need to identify additional immunosuppressants for use in transplantation, specifically compounds that are simultaneously Treg-protective and capable of blocking memory T cells."[106]

With guidance from Dr. Heeger, Dr. Reid-Adam and her coresearchers screened extracts from 53 traditional Chinese herbs for their ability to suppress human alloreactive T cells (T cells mobilized by the presence of transplanted tissue). The team reasoned that herbs would ideally inhibit production of the proinflammatory cytokine IFN-γ and simultaneously augment production of the immunoregulatory cytokine IL-10. Says Reid-Adam, "An increase in IFN-γ is good for allergies but bad for organ rejection. However, IL-10, which sometimes indicates greater Th2 activity but not really Th1, can be a beneficial indicator for allergies and also good for transplantation."

Employing an *in vitro* version of transplantation—culturing cells from one individual and then exposing those to cells from another—they analyzed the cytokines in the presence of each herb, using the standard low-dose–high-dose protocol.

They identified *Qu Mai* (QM, *Dianthus superbus*), a member of the carnation family, as a candidate. Dr. Reid-Adam says, "There isn't much written about it in Western literature, but TCM practitioners use it to treat blood in urine and urinary infection, indicating a connection to the kidney, and for skin inflammation. It achieves the decrease in an important proinflammatory cytokine without killing immune cells." Testing in paired doses they found that the higher the dose, the greater improvement in the ratio of IL-10 to IFN- .

Further research based on polarity isolated three fractions of active compounds from the QM herbal preparation. These were dichloromethane-soluble QMAD (mainly contains nonpolar compounds), ethyl acetate-soluble QMAE (mainly contains less polar compounds), and butanol-soluble QMAB (mainly contains moderate polar compounds). Testing each fraction for its effects on cytokine pro-duction showed that the QMAD fraction induced the most favorable effects, yielding a nine-fold increase in IL-10:IFN-g ratios

The QMAD data show an additional benefit over conventional immunosuppressants, which show limited ability to modulate the memory T cells. This in effect keeps the immune system in a state of continuous emergency as long as the foreign tissue remains in the body. The "data show unequivocal effects of QMAD on inhibiting proliferation and IFN-γ production by naïve and memory T cells while simultaneously facilitating Treg induction. The observed ability of QMAD to block proliferation and cytokine secretion by memory T cells is of particular interest, as memory T cells are generally resistant to immunosuppression and have been implicated as key mediators of allograft* injury." If this pans out in subsequent research, it will ease some of the perpetual struggle between the patient's own immune system and the new organ, possibly prolonging the life of each transplanted kidney and improving the patient's quality of life.

---

* "Allograft: The transplant of an organ or tissue from one individual to another of the same species with a different genotype. For example, a transplant from one person to another, but not an identical twin, is an allograft. Allografts account for many human transplants, including those from cadaveric, living related, and living unrelated donors" (MedicineNet.com).

Two cautionary notes: As Dr. Cullen points out, favorable test-tube results do not guarantee clinical efficacy, and unlike FAHF-2, Dr. Reid-Adam's work is not likely to lead to a "cure." Assuming QM proves itself in animal models, the population of human subjects whose kidneys are failing can't submit to placebo-controlled trials or be left untreated to test lasting efficacy.

"I see it as adjunctive," Dr. Reid-Adam says. "Anything that can provide relief and mitigate damage from general immune suppression will be a great step forward."

Asthma

Dollar for dollar, and life for life, asthma poses the largest challenge to American public health, and indeed around the world, of any allergic disease. As discussed in chapter 1, asthma takes more than 3000 lives every year, including almost 200 children under the age of 15.[107] The medical costs and indirect costs such as lost productivity at work and at school come to $56 billion annually. Per capita, the burden is even worse in many other countries, including, notably, New Zealand, Australia, and the United Kingdom.

In all these countries, however, mortality rates have fallen considerably with the use of inhaled corticosteroids (ICS) the biggest factor in improvement. Still, many of the continuing deaths are considered preventable, if only more patients were compliant with their medication regimes. Apart from the cost of medication and the day-to-day aggravation of taking medicine, the negative associations with the word "steroids" in the name is a major barrier, although corticosteroids have no connection to the testosterone-based steroids that athletes use.

ASHMI, described in the previous chapter, may present an effective alternative to ICS. In an early double-blind, randomized, placebo-controlled trial investigating the efficacy and tolerability of ASHMI compared with oral prednisone therapy in 91 patients with moderate-to-severe asthma, treatment was administered daily over 4 weeks.[108] After treatment, lung function was significantly improved in both groups, and clinical symptom scores, use of bronchodilators, and serum IgE levels and Th2 cytokine levels were reduced. Unlike prednisone, ASHMI significantly increased serum IFN-γ and cortisol levels while no significant side effects were observed. (Cortisol is the body's own cortisone, which helps mitigate allergic activity.) Subsequent experiments affirmed safety and tolerance, as well as favorable intermodulatory effects on cytokines, IgE levels, and bronchoconstriction.[109]

> Taken together these studies showed that ASHMI was safe and well tolerated in clinical study. ASHMI also showed multiple beneficial effects in allergic asthma. Because ASHMI enhanced IFN-γ, and normalized cortisol levels in a clinical study, future clinical investigations should determine if ASHMI can restore/normal IFN-γ and cortisol levels when used in combination with corticosteroids. Identification of active compounds in ASHMI will enhance our understanding of the pharmacological mechanisms of ASHMI and may lead to novel drugs for asthma therapy.[110]

(ASHMI is not the only TCM-derived asthma treatment under study. A more complete discussion is available in the review article cited above.)

Dr. Li already uses ASHMI in her clinic, where it is used as a supplement rather than a drug. "We have to be careful," she says. "Our eczema treatment can start on day one. With steroids, you can't just suddenly stop and switch to something new because inflammation may return while the new treatment takes hold. We introduce the new treatment and taper off the steroids. The whole time, we keep records on IgE levels and lung function, which confirm what we are seeing in our clinical trials. That is, ASHMI has clinical efficacy."

Cancer

No discussion of the capacity of herbal medicine to modulate the immune system (or excite the world about the possibilities) would be complete without including cancer. In 1971, President Richard Nixon signed the National Cancer Act, also known as the "War on Cancer." Trillions of dollars have been spent to fund basic research on the molecular mechanisms behind cell division and their regulation. Trillions more have been spent on treatments, but cancer remains a tremendous drain on patient health and finances. As I am writing this, the *New York Times* (April 24, 2013) carries a story Doctors Denounce Cancer Drug Prices of $100,000 a Year, which explains that "more than 100 influential cancer specialists from around the world have taken the unusual step of banding together in hopes of persuading some leading pharmaceutical companies to bring prices down."

Maybe it didn't have to be this way. There was a point more than a century ago when the industrial model of cancer treatment was paralleled by research on the immune system. In 2012, Dr. Jerome Groopman published an article in *The New Yorker* called "The T-Cell Army,"[111] which tells the story of a New York surgeon named William Coley who lost a patient, Elizabeth Dashiell, to sarcoma in 1891 and devoted himself to finding a cure. In the records of New York Hospital,

> He found one patient who stood out from the grim stories. Eleven years earlier, Fred Stein, a German immigrant who worked as a housepainter, had a rapidly growing sarcoma in his neck. After four operations and four recurrences of the cancer, a senior surgeon declared Stein's case "absolutely hopeless." Then an infection caused by streptococcal bacteria broke out in red patches across Stein's neck and face. There were no antibiotics at the time, so his immune system was left to fight off the infection unaided. Remarkably, as his white blood cells combatted the bacteria, the sarcoma shrank into a bland scar. Stein left the hospital with no infection and no discernible cancer. Coley concluded that something in Stein's own body had shrunk the cancer.

Groopman tells us that for a decade, Coley pursued the hypothesis that the immune system could be harnessed for cancer, which one colleague called "whispers of nature," supported by John D. Rockefeller, who had been personally close to the deceased Miss Dashiell. At the same time, Rockefeller was backing the work of Dr. James Ewing, who thought that the newly discovered miracle of radiation was the only treatment for cancer. The Rockefeller family's interest in cancer treatment had begun with John D.'s father, "Doctor William A. Rockefeller, the Celebrated Cancer Specialist," who sold a treatment made of—what else?—the crude oil that provided the basis for the family fortune.[112]

Eventually, Rockefeller threw his money behind the industrial model that led to our current reliance on radiation and chemotherapy, whose side effects are so dire that they sound like the medical version of the Vietnam War pronouncement "We had to destroy the village in order to save it."

Now, however, there is a resurgence of interest in exploring the possibility of using the immune system for cancer. In the months since Groopman's *New Yorker* piece came out, the *New York Times* has published several articles. One was about Dr. Ralph Steinman, who tried "to concoct a set of treatments from his body's own ingredients, which could take over from his chemotherapy and form a customized, dynamic treatment for his disease." [113] Dr. Steinman died several hours before he was to be informed that he would be sharing a Nobel Prize, which put the award in doubt, because it's not to be given posthumously (an exception was made).

Another *Times* article was about the work of Dr. Suzanne L. Topalian, a melanoma specialist at Johns Hopkins University, on a drug to thwart a "molecular shield" that protects tumors from attacks by the immune system. [114]

A third tells of a young leukemia patient who was given a disabled HIV virus that reprogrammed her immune system to fight the cancer. [115]

Thus, we come to the potential of ASHMI for fighting cancer. A colleague of Dr. Li, Martin J. Walsh, PhD, Associate Professor of Structural and Chemical Biology, Pediatrics, Hepatology, and Genetics and Genomic Sciences, has investigated the possibilities in the laboratory in collaboration with Dr. Li.[116] He writes in the Abstract of an unpublished article called Inhibition of Tumor Cell Growth by Herbal Preparation MSSM-03:

> The use of herbal medicine has been in use over several centuries with little known about either the biochemical basis or genetic mechanisms that regulate the actions of herbal medicine. Since the efficacy and safety profile of many herbal preparations have been unofficially validated, more government focus on the use of these medicinal products has allowed their use to be more widely accepted by the medical community at large with legal provisions for their use. Because of the pleiotropic [producing more than one effect] actions of herbal medicine to direct broad activities over the host organism, it is likely that herbal medicines are comprised of several unknown bioactive compounds that interact with several signaling pathways.

Walsh and his colleagues studied ASHMI—MSSM-03, which is its name for purposes of research at Mount Sinai School of Medicine—for its potential to suppress growth of tumor cells in culture. Using immunoblot analysis of tumor cells treated with MSSM-03, they found that after 18 hours, the proteins in tumor cells that inhibit growth increased, while those that encourage growth had separated into harmless components. They add, "These studies provide evidence that MSSM-03 is a tumor cell growth inhibitor and may indicate potential use in treatment of hyperplastic growth diseases, such as cancer."

15.

Treating Severe Allergic Diseases:
Three Cases from Private Clinical Practice

While Dr. Xiu-Min Li is an extraordinary scientist, she is also a great clinical practitioner, a healer. As Scott Sicherer says, in China, TCM is just medicine.

Dr. Li employs a much larger array of compounds at her private practice than are currently being studied. The medications qualify for use with patients as supplements with a long history of safe use and, as employed under Xiu-Min's standards, nontoxicity, although they are not reimbursable by insurance companies.

She introduced me to three families who have benefited from her treatments from among the dozens who have passed through her doors from states across this country, as well as from the United Kingdom, Spain, Canada, Australia, France, and India. Having spent the best part of this book explaining how these treatments work in theory, I also want you to see why Xiu-Min's faith in their efficacy is well founded, although these accounts qualify as anecdotal evidence, not scientifically verified. However Chinese doctors have arrived at their formulas and strategies over the centuries, those formulas and strategies do seem to work. I also wanted to share these stories because they point the way toward incorporating these treatments into Western clinical practice, Dr. Li's dream of integrative medicine.

Julie

Dr. Elena Simon (name changed) is an emergency room doctor at a community hospital two hours from Toronto who occasionally works shifts as long as 36 hours, depending on the availability of other doctors. She says that until the age of 14, her daughter Julie was an outgoing straight-A student and cheerleader with no health issues to speak of. One night three years ago, while out for dinner at a Thai restaurant with her father, Julie's life changed. She began to break out in hives, and her throat began to tighten. Her father took her to an emergency room—not the one where Elena works—where she was treated for anaphylaxis.

The local allergist tested Julie for allergies to peanut and tree nuts—staples of Thai cooking—but nothing stood out. Over the next several weeks, this scenario played out repeatedly, fortunately with three-hour delayed onset so there was sufficient time to react medically. With no adequate answers available in their rural community, the next stop was the Hospital for Sick Children in Toronto, (referred to by doctors as "Sick Kids"), where Elena had done part of her training in family medicine. Sick Kids has an allergy department, although there was no treatment in the hospital except to give epinephrine and antihistamines.

Julie became so reactive that she would react to trace allergens in her nut-free school. She couldn't walk through a grocery store without responding, and she ended up in the Toronto ER an average of every two weeks. After a lifetime as a star student, her repeated absences took a toll on her schoolwork. All told, Julie missed half a year of school over the next two years. "She spent so much time in the emergency room hooked up to IVs that she was on a first-name basis with the entire staff. Whenever she returned, the ER nurses and doctors would say, 'You again.'" Dr. Simon's own work began to suffer as well, as she was forced to deal with repeated emergencies and to provide homeschooling.

Elena told me, "Obviously, we couldn't go on like this. I began to suffer physically and emotionally, too. I'm a doctor, but I'm a mother first. But my problems were nothing compared to my daughter's. She became depressed for the first time in her life. She was put on prednisone and became moon-faced [a physical symptom of prolonged use of systemic steroids] and even suicidal." A full-blown psychotic breakdown that required a late-night two-hour drive to Toronto was attributed to the prednisone, and the doctors took Julie off it. The head of psychiatry, a friend of Dr. Simon's at Sick Kids, said he had never seen anything like it. Removing the steroids improved Julie's state of mind but put her at greater risk of anaphylaxis.

The low point came when Julie went on an overnight camping trip on an island with her classmates, which is a traditional rite of passage for her school. Her mom gave her four EpiPens as well as antihistamines to take with her—and still, she had anaphylaxis. The helicopter ambulance couldn't land, so she had to be ferried to the opposite shore by canoe and put aboard an ambulance—at which point she had already used three EpiPens—all this in the middle of the night lighted by spotlights from the helicopter!

At last, Dr. Simon read about Dr. Li and FAHF-2. She made an appointment at Dr. Li's New York private clinic, where both mother and daughter acquired an instant sense of hope. "She was so warm and welcoming, and talked with us for two hours taking a full medical history. I believe in bedside manner, and I have never seen anything like this. She even gave Julie an acupuncture treatment."

Then began a regimen of 50 pills a day. Within 6 months, Julie had no hives at all and no constriction of her throat. Where she had been taking so much Benadryl that she was sleepy all the time, followed by a period in which it lost its sedating effects altogether, Julie has only taken two Benadryl in months for one minor reaction. She went back in school and graduated on time.

After a year on the treatment, life is now so normal that Julie is back to being a teenager, and impatient with the continued daily dosing, but Dr. Simon insists. "She has her life back. And Dr. Li is my medical hero."

Postscript from Dr. Simon: "Julie was just away in France taking a course this past month. Amazingly, she encountered nuts accidentally in a pastry and did not react. Then, she did not tell me but stopped taking the medicine while she was there and ate many nuts in pastries, including almonds, which she was very allergic to, and was fine! When she returned, she also ate a chocolate spread with mixed nuts in it in front of me, which she did not react to at all. She wants to continue without the medicine and see how things go. I almost cannot believe my eyes. She has been on the protocol for a year, taking it religiously."

Jackie

Jackie O. is a 10-year-old girl allergic to eggs, peanuts, fish, seeds, citrus fruits, and nuts, with a history of anaphylaxis, asthma, and total blood IgE of 6000. Although most allergists don't consider blood IgE levels as confirmation of food allergy on their own (history of reactivity is the surest sign), anything over 100 is considered high, and much lower levels do not preclude dangerous reactions. Levels as high as 6000 are indicative of serious allergies.

Although multiple food allergies were a big issue for Jackie, as they are for millions of others, the more immediate problem was that she suffered from severe intractable eczema. "It was everywhere," Jackie says, "my face, my neck, my eyelids, and down to my feet."

Her father, Greg, said to me, "It's terrible that an eight-year-old girl could be so self-conscious that she didn't want to go to school." Peer judgment aside, Jackie's teachers noticed her discomfort and were continually asking if she was all right.

She couldn't sleep through the night. "I used to wake up crying in the night. My friends thought I had polka-dot sheets because they had blood from scratching."

Says her father, "It was a big negative feedback loop. Lack of sleep weakened her immune system, leaving her vulnerable to other infections."

Jackie's allergist, who happened to be my cousin, Dr. Paul Ehrlich, tried all the conventional treatments: antihistamines, steroidal creams, and gauze wraps to protect her skin from scratching fingers. "I looked like a mummy," says Jackie. Nothing worked. And then Paul did the New York equivalent of sending her to Lourdes. He referred her to Dr. Li's private clinic.

The first session consisted of a couple of hours of talk with Mom and Dad present, ending with Dr. Li's pronouncement, "I will try to help you." With the second session began a daily regimen of a special herbal soaking bath, and five kinds of capsules totaling 64 (which Jackie could not swallow so instead made them into a hot tea), and a nightly rub with a black cream called IABZC everywhere below the neck, waiting for five minutes before putting on her pajamas. Eventually she was able to swallow the capsules instead of making them into tea, and currently she is down to "just" 38 per day.

Within a month and a half, Jackie started to improve rapidly. "It was night and day," says her father. Jackie's teachers began to notice that the redness was going away and couldn't help commenting. Jackie's asthma was also better. After a bit more than two years of treatment, Jackie's skin is so normal that she has to be reminded as she's going out the door for school in the morning to take her pills, which she finds as disgusting as the tea, and she faces two to three more years of treatment.

Paul follows up on Jackie's IgE levels and her liver and kidney function annually. Her total IgE went down from ~6000 to ~3000 after one year of treatment and to ~1800 after two years of treatment. Peanut IgE reduced about tenfold (from ~30 to 3); tree nut, fish, and sesame IgE levels also went down. Jackie's liver and kidney function are all in normal range.

Her father says, "How can these ingredients I can't pronounce make her so much better?"

Jackie can pronounce the name of Dr. Li's herbal medicines. She gave Dr. Li a gift, which is a drawing in Chinese characters meaning "harmony" and "hope." Jackie says of Dr. Li, "She changed my life. Without her, I wouldn't be sitting here with a smile on my face."

The story gets better. After a few months of treatment, Dr. Li approved more strenuous aerobic activity to strengthen Jackie's lungs. Jackie has been riding a two-wheeler since she was four with her dad every chance she got and at age nine joined the children's cycling team Star Track in NYC. After a year of treatment, her asthma had improved so much that she won several local races as well as the New York State Championship for her age division. This gave her enough confidence to set a goal for the 2013 Junior National Championships. In July of 2013, as the second youngest competitor in the girl's 10–12 division, she finished 17th in the time trial and 15th in the road race and promptly crowned herself "fastest 10-year-old female cyclist in the US." "It was such a major victory for her just to be there," her dad said. "To think where she was two and a half years ago, and now she is competing against the best girls her age in the country is nothing short of a miracle."

Aaron

Aaron (name changed) was a colicky baby. As he began eating solids at the age of six months, he started projectile vomiting frequently, but without pattern. The pediatrician recommended scaling back his diet to breast milk and rice cereal. Foods were reintroduced and new foods were introduced without any problems for a few weeks. The cycle soon would soon begin again, however, so Aaron's parents would scale back to the basics, then reintroduce other food, and again, the roller coaster would start. The pediatrician didn't have any answers.

Kate, Aaron's mother, took the 10-month-old boy to see a pediatric gastroenterologist who suggested that the problem might be celiac disease (an immune reaction to gluten, a protein in wheat, barley, and rye) or possibly food allergies. The doctor tested Aaron, who had 3 of the 4 markers for celiac, and wanted to "scope" him (pass an endoscope through his mouth and stomach to take a tissue sample from his small intestine). Anxious to spare their son the trauma, however, Aaron's parents took him for a second opinion at Miami Children's Hospital, where the GI specialist recommended against it.

Aaron was also referred to an allergist who conducted RASTs, which showed sensitivity to eight foods. The allergist told Kate to keep all of these foods out of the boy's diet, despite the fact that on many days, he would eat the foods and not have any allergic reaction. Kate tried the elimination diet. Aaron experienced hives at 12 months after consuming dairy and at 15 months after consuming baked egg whites.

The vomiting cycle continued. When Aaron was 12 months old, the pediatrician prescribed Zantac, an anti-reflux medicine, for a year, which seemed to help as the vomiting episodes subsided.

Eating at restaurants wasn't much of a problem because there were many restaurants that were kosher for either meat or dairy. As Aaron's family learned, however, there is a difference between *parve*—dairy free for religious purposes, which is determined by weight—and completely dairy *protein*-free. Still, kosher restaurants that served meat did provide some leeway. Even this was not enough, however, when two-year-old Aaron began playing with hummus that was served instead of butter with bread on the tables and reacted to the sesame it contained. Other foods provoked hives, facial swelling, and vomiting.

Aaron's food and environmental allergen list grew, and more things were dropped from his diet. The doctors projected that he might outgrow his allergies by age 3, then 5, then 8, and 10. Aaron had trouble gaining weight and growing. He came home early from school regularly because of allergic reactions to food in science experiments and in special treats. Aaron's throat became itchy just being near the popcorn popped in the school courtyard as a Friday-afternoon treat. Kate added accommodations to Aaron's "504 plan," which refers to Section 504 of the Rehabilitation Act and the Americans with Disabilities Act, specifying that no one with a disability can be excluded from participating in federally funded programs or activities at school. No science experiment dealing with food could include any of his allergens; a week's notice of any activities involving food must be given to Kate so she could help protect her son.

Allergy shots were initiated for Aaron's environmental allergens, but the big problem was eating. At 9 years old, he was having problems again with intermittent vomiting and diarrhea, except it was worse this time. He couldn't keep food or liquid down, and after each vomiting episode, he remained lethargic for a day or two. After a trip to the ER for dehydration (and during which he could not take the hospital's anti-vomiting medication because the inactive ingredients included an allergen), he saw another gastroenterologist.

Eventually, Aaron was diagnosed with EoE, an allergic condition mediated not by mast cells but other effector cells called eosinophils that show up where they don't belong. These reactions can be delayed 12 to 48 hours after exposure to an allergen, possibly, as new research shows,[117] because they are triggered by basophils, the effector cells associated with late-phase IgE-mediated allergies. Day-to-day existence became, in Kate's words, "a fine line between quality of life and sustenance." The wrong foods would result in hours of vomiting and diarrhea, followed by 24–48 hours of lethargy. At age 11, Aaron weighed just 59 pounds.

Disappointed by conventional treatment, Kate began researching alternatives, including OIT and FAHF-2 trials, but EoE was disqualifying for all those. However, Kate brought Aaron to see Dr. Li in her private clinic, where he received a regimen of herbal medications to reduce his eosinophils and allergic reactions. The medication regimen includes *Mei Huang* Tea III pills, Digestive Tea capsules, *Xuo Xiang Zheng Qi Wan* pills, Seasonal Herbal Capsules, bath additives, and skin creams. After 6 months, Aaron was asymptomatic and his eczema had improved.

A year after treatment commenced, the differences in Aaron's health and quality of life were "night and day," according to his mother. He gained weight. His breathing was much better, particularly at night. His eosinophil count, although still high at 69, was down from 225. Aaron's reactions grew milder and milder. A reaction on January 8, 2013, at 8:30 AM—thought to be a delayed reaction—was so mild that he was in school at 11:30. He had no other reactions until June when he reacted 36 hours after a baked egg challenge. In July, he passed a pecan challenge. Outside the immediate family, the person most deeply impressed by Aaron's improvement was the school nurse. Her job was much less frantic in the last six months of the school year because Aaron was no longer a frequent visitor.

16

The Slow Road to Clinical Practice

The earliest publications of Dr. Li's research that have led to the clinical trials now underway are almost 20 years old, with more years of research still to come. The journey to clinical practice is not just a matter of research, however. There are also matters of culture and custom, both for patients and for doctors.

Will people accept these therapies? Judging by the numbers of patients who have sought CAM treatments (see chapter 1), the demand side is already there. Anxious parents are clearly clamoring for results. This is why, after all, what we might call an OIT underground has sprung up, not to mention many treatments that have their origins in what we might call the web-footed school of medicine.

The question then becomes who will provide these treatments. Will physicians adopt new medications that come from outside the pharmaceutical mainstream? Dr. Lisa Sanders has written, "Doctors are not known for their rapid embrace of the new....Physicians are so reluctant to change the way they practice medicine that it takes an average seventeen years for techniques well established by research—such as giving an aspirin to a patient having a heart attack—to be adopted by even half of those in practice."[118] In his book *How Doctors Think*, Dr. Jerome Groopman cites Douglas Watson, former president and CEO of Novartis, to the effect that research shows that most physicians regularly prescribe around two dozen drugs, most of which they learned about during their training, although their training may have taken place many years earlier.[119] I have no reason to think it's any different with allergists. *

Dr. Renata Engler of Walter Reed National Military Medical Center is one of Dr. Li's greatest admirers. She described the dimensions of the challenge in a 2000 article about Dr. Li's early research:

> The scope of what is included in the array of CAM treatments can be overwhelming to the health care providers trying to learn about them. Herbal medicine alone encompasses several textbooks of information but with no well-defined "evidence-based" guidelines or easily accessed educational material. Most physicians complain of difficulty remaining current with the knowledge required for the practice of allopathic medicine. Therapeutic arenas such as herbal medicine (with more than 1800 herbals currently available on the US market) are overwhelming in informational content. It has been easier to ignore the whole area of CAM as "placebo" or "not effective" and many patients complain that it is difficult to find a health care provider willing to partner with alternative practitioners or to monitor them if they choose an herbal or other CAM therapeutic trial outside the Food and Drug Administration–approved pharmaceutical industry." P. 628

Thirteen years later, Dr. Engler remains skeptical about mainstream allergy practice meeting patient needs, and about practitioners' receptivity to CAM. She told me, "The system is currently failing a lot of patients. There's a tendency to abandon those who don't fit into comfortable evidence-based slots. This includes a high percentage of asthma cases and food-allergy patients. Our community consigns patients to hopelessness or treatments that are worse than the disease. Steroids haven't answered the mail for everyone."

---

* The one potentially game-changing tool I am familiar with is component testing, which helps establish which components of allergenic proteins a person reacts to, and can help predict the severity of allergic reactions, although it is nowhere near definitive. Years after component testing's FDA approval, many allergists continue to rely on testing technology that is widely acknowledged to be obsolete. (I must point out that I was paid by the manufacturer, ThermoFisherScientific *all too briefly* several years go to supply news items for its consumer blog. I continue to talk with the company's personnel regularly because they still represent the cutting edge in testing.)

Engler also blames the high-altitude perspective of certain regulators who control the financial spigot, citing a colleague whose funding was turned off because the decision makers were no longer interested in "individual patients." Her critique extends to the national research agenda: "Fifty percent of evidence-based medicine is significantly revised and/or reversed in five years. Most money goes into confirming what we already know instead of focusing on the gaps where we could add information."

However, other regulators show signs of a more expansive attitude toward alternatives. Acupuncture needles have been recognized as medical devices, and health insurance often covers part of the cost of treatment. Dr. Li says, "Current methodology of clinical trials does not totally fit the nature of traditional Chinese medicine, which is a more personalized medicine. The NIH encourages investigators to develop a more sophisticated methodology for clinical studies of complementary and alternative medicines."

According to Dr. Li, FAHF-2 faces 8 to 10 more years of clinical trials (and tens of millions of dollars) before it will qualify as a pharmaceutical that can be reimbursable under current FDA standards and prescribed by practicing allergists with no special training. She says, "The FDA has issued guidance for botanical drug investigation. Some herbal medicines may be classified as prescription drugs after completing the clinical trials." The current state of regulation with Dr. Li's unique circumstances does offer an intermediate road to treatment, however.

For one thing, some traditional Chinese medicines are already cleared for use as "dietary supplements." For another, they have a track record. Traditional Chinese medicines are regulated as medicines in China, Japan, and Korea, where they are part of mainstream medical care, are prescribed by doctors, and are dispensed in hospital pharmacies. They can also be used as over-the-counter medicines. Australia has also endorsed the use of some classical medicines based on a long history of safe and effective use. Finally, the medicines that Dr. Li uses already pass the most rigorous standards for safety and purity in the world, based on their certification both in China and at the lab at Mount Sinai.

Given the ineffectiveness of current practice at treating food allergies, I have a feeling that if there were a food-allergy pill today, many allergists would prescribe it, if only because they have so few options. Some doctors are openly frustrated at the limitations of today's medicine. I heard Dr. John Oppenheimer of New Jersey, who has had a distinguished career in both allergy research and practice, lament the fact that he often felt more like a risk manager than a healer.

Dr. Anna Nowak-Wegzryn, Dr. Li's colleague at Mount Sinai, told me that the fact that FAHF-2 is botanical in origin and has the aura of alternative medicine around it wouldn't be an impediment: "We use botanical-based drugs all the time." Surveys also show that, all things being equal, patients and their parents would prefer "natural" remedies to synthetic ones.

Certainly, I don't expect that allergists, even newly minted ones, will achieve grounding in alternative and complementary medicine any time soon. Allergy fellows (and there aren't a lot of them) learn from older doctors (few of whom, if any, have the necessary background).

Dr. Engler and several colleagues described the challenge of acquiring the necessary expertise in their aptly named article "Complementary and Alternative Medicine for the Allergist-Immunologist: Where Do I Start?"[120] They say,

> Allergy-immunology specialists are faced with the challenge of how to respond practically to the evolving information presented by the expanding world of CAM. The spectrum of positions on CAM within conventional medical practices ranges from "don't ask, don't tell" to establishing a partnership with the patient who may be seeking or is already using CAM therapies. A small percentage of practitioners are incorporating both conventional and nontraditional medical therapies, reflecting a movement toward integrative medicine. Many physicians and health care workers in general are interested in learning more about CAM but are overwhelmed by the amount of information and afraid of entering into any discussions with their patients because of a possible liability risk and/or time requirement. p. 310

Furthermore, Dr. Engler and her coauthors point out that the magnitude of new information to assimilate on top of what they already know is daunting:

> The key elements of physician-patient interactions that involve CAM questions and/or therapeutic impact include the following: (1) exploring factors driving interest in CAM; (2) documenting clinical reasons for

seeking CAM options; (3) assessing current dis-
ease/health status and therapies to date; (4) documenting patient's preferences and reasons; (5)
assessing and documenting adequacy of medical evaluation; (6) defining a plan for follow-up visits; (7) providing good risk communications with option for
additional consultative visits; (8) acknowledging
evolving expectations and goals; (9) educating about
new safety and/or efficacy issues related to CAM
choices during each visit; and (10) addressing need for
further consultations and how these consultations can
be optimized.

How can this synthesis of alternative and mainstream treatment be achieved without burdening a dwindling pool of allergists with an additional fellowship in the middle or end of an established career? (By the way, they have plenty to keep them busy between the 40-yard lines of standard allergy care.)

Thus came Dr. Li's vision of a "Center for Integrative Medicine for Allergies and Wellness." The idea of integrative medicine is popular now. Memorial Sloan Kettering Cancer Center offers services to "complement mainstream cancer care [including] touch therapy, mind-body therapy, acupuncture, creative therapy, and nutrition counseling, as well as exercise programs to improve strength and promote relaxation." Many of these elements have analogues in TCM, and indeed, some of them are derived from it. The biggest difference between the Sloan Kettering model and Dr. Li's vision is that hers carries with it a pharmacopeia to treat disease, not just to enhance patients' overall health while they endure chemotherapy and radiation.

Furthering the synthesis of TCM with Western medicine, which is called "translational research," Dr. Li's center will bridge the two worlds of medicine both for science and for treatment.

The parallel tracks of pioneering research and active current clinical practice give Dr. Li a unique advantage. For one thing, the fact that she works with therapies similar to those that are already available by prescription in China and Japan gives the medicines created under her supervision a leg up in the US approval process. Her private practice has grown without any Web presence or advertising. She started it because she wanted to provide an option for the families and patients who are interested in TCM but weren't qualified for or didn't want to take part in trials. She says,

> In general, the patients and families find me though a referral from my colleagues at Mount Sinai, or other pediatricians, allergists, and dermatologists as well as the families. Family referral is becoming more common now. For example, after I see the first member of the family then other members start coming, too. Usually I see the children first and then the parents. This is because family history is important to allergy. In addition, some people find me though the publications from my group.

The second reason that Dr. Li's unique circumstances offer an intermediate road to treatment is that her private clinic provides a real-world context for study, which is often lacking with allergy-related research. Asthma trials, for example, have been explicitly criticized for being optimized to study conditions using a more homogeneous study population than would be likely to take the medicine, and producing results that are far more favorable than those obtained in actual patient use.[121] Dr. Li's private practice can encompass patients with a greater variety of conditions and ages. (Whatever their variations, however, all patients are required to be tested for IgE, liver function, and other measures to ensure that their data can be incorporated into larger studies.)

Even before Dr. Li's new center gets off the ground, however, she and her colleagues have improvised several models for extending her ideas into mainstream treatment. For one thing, the medical school students at Mount Sinai established an integrative-medicine club. Medical students and interns are spending their summer in her labs, doing research and helping draft case report manuscripts based on unique cases. Likewise, clinical fellows are continually doing research in her lab.

Dr. Li has also begun a pilot program at the initiative of an asthma specialist in California who wrote to her because he has a number of patients who do not respond to inhaled corticosteroids or omalizumab. They have agreed that the California doctor will supply detailed histories and measurements for these patients and Dr. Li will provide the medications and the strategies for treatment, which will be delivered locally but supervised by her at a distance.

Another integrative approach sprang from treatment of a young man with a history of eczema, asthma, food allergies, and environmental allergies. His mother wanted to have his environmental allergies treated by her local allergist with SLIT, an alternative to allergy shots. To avoid the risk that SLIT allergens would aggravate his eczema and asthma, they chose to attack these conditions through use of TCM as well as treatment of his food allergies. The two doctors have developed a collaborative relationship, and the mother is pleased enough with the results for her son thus far to volunteer to help raise funds for the next phase of research using B-FAHF-2.

Still another approach for bridging alternative and mainstream practice is for Dr. Li to mentor mainstream practitioners as an extension of her private clinical practice. She has reached out to a select set of allergists in New York with a set of parameters of the patients she wants to treat collaboratively, basically the "worst of the worst" cases. She says, "These are people who have nowhere else to turn." A history of severe food allergy reactions or an additional symptom such as bad asthma is considered off limits for most clinical trials.

Dr. Li has outlined a set of specific parameters for these referrals. What they have in common are proven links to other conditions that are taking a discernible toll on the patients' quality of life. Improvement in these conditions serves as a marker for improvement in the underlying allergies. The parameters are listed below. (If they sound familiar, it is because they echo the kinds of comorbid illnesses described, and successfully treated, in the previous chapter.)

1. ***Recalcitrant eczema associated with food allergy, with total IgE greater than 2000 and elevated peanut-specific IgE.*** The reasons for this parameter are several. First, patients with levels that high are out of bounds even for other new treatments, let alone conventional ones. Peanut allergy might respond to anti-IgE therapy (omalizumab, or Xolair), although it is not currently approved for that purpose, but in any case, it does not work well or is not recommended for someone with IgE levels above 2000. Second, as already discussed, patients outgrow peanut allergies only 20% of the time and have the most to gain. Third, peanut-allergic children with intractable eczema have persistently high rates of peanut-specific IgE even when they conscientiously avoid the allergen.

2. *Frequent reactions associated with food allergy that severely compromise patients' quality of life.* As the case of Julie in the previous chapter shows, food-allergy reactions can take over the life of a previously highly functioning patient. The continuous threat of reaction can result in anxiety levels so high that it becomes impossible to distinguish between *actual* exposure to allergens and *perceived* exposure. Even in clinical trials, anxiety can run so high that it occasionally becomes necessary to administer epinephrine when the patient has received a placebo. In these cases, the holistic model of treatment characteristic of TCM serves several purposes simultaneously, gaining the patient's trust to minimize anxiety while treating both the underlying immune disorders and the symptoms. In mainstream treatment, the psychology is often treated separately.

3. *Symptomatic EoE.* This is a big one for many reasons. It is one of a number of so-called mixed-type mediated food disorders. Sixty percent of EoE patients also have positive serum IgE to foods, according to the 2010 NIAID food allergy guidelines.[122] EoE is a relatively new allergic disease. It was not even mentioned in my copy of the *Atlas of Allergic Diseases*, which was published in 2002—eosinophilic gastritis, yes, EoE no.[123] The standard treatment is that frustrating combination of avoidance and steroids.[124] Aaron's case in the previous chapter was typical: He had both IgE-mediated food allergies and EoE. He was a typical patient: young and male, and subject to delayed-onset long-lasting symptoms that frequently result in failure to thrive. EoE is an automatic disqualifier for OIT in clinical trials and OIT offered by private practitioners for a very good reason: Doses of the allergen will provoke unpleasant symptoms of another disease.

4. *Symptomatic asthma/allergic rhinitis that can be treated along with food allergies.* Day by day, asthma and allergic rhinitis make patients more miserable than food allergies do, provided, of course, the food allergies are controlled through avoidance. The threat of food allergies is demoralizing; the realities of asthma and allergic rhinitis are

depressing, distracting, and conspicuous. These other allergic diseases are so much as part of everyday life that improvement can provide a significant marker for measuring the progress of fixing the immune system overall. Nasal symptoms and breathing will improve as the IgE mechanism is modulated toward normal.

All the above conditions have both objective and subjective outcomes. Patients who perceive improvement in their quality of life will be most likely to persevere while waiting for the more abstract benefits of food-allergy therapy take hold. Collaboration with the primary allergists to add complementary therapy will reinforce compliance while also transferring knowledge of a new and hopeful approach to an intractable problem.

Missing from this list of priority patients are those whose food allergies are well controlled because they are disciplined in their avoidance and for whom the sole monitoring tool is allergen-specific IgE in the blood. As mentioned, IgE is a poor indicator for clinical allergy. Some patients with relatively low blood IgE levels can experience anaphylaxis from minor exposures, whereas others with much higher levels can eat a food safely. For patients who have food allergies but no co-morbid allergies that can stand in for measuring treatment progress, Dr. Li is working on a more direct route to safety. She says,

> We have identified several compounds from FAHF-2 and ASHMI that directly suppress IgE. Beyond FAHF-2 and ASHMI, we have built up an inventory of more than 1000 TCMs at our lab. We used IgE-producing B-cell lines to screen the medicines with most potent IgE inhibitory effects and identify the active compounds. We have found two compounds that were very potent and safe in direct suppression of B-cell IgE production. My goal is a more potent and convenient natural treatment that reduces IgE quickly while still being very safe.

It must also be pointed out that for the time being, patients who visit the clinic will have to be sufficiently well off to afford these treatments, although the treatments are comparable in price to the OIT that many families are paying for out of pocket and to the combination of health care cost and income loss incurred by parents' sacrifice to help manage food allergies (chapter 1).

The parameters have now been shared with a select number of New York allergists, spearheaded by my cousin, Dr. Paul Ehrlich, who is perennially one of the top pediatric allergists in New York and past president of the New York Allergy and Asthma Society. Patients will be treated both by their own allergists and Dr. Li, and in the process, some of her approach will be shared with the mainstream doctors.

Dr. Li doesn't expect the mainstream physicians to become TCM doctors. "Younger physicians will be able to go further," she says. "Allergists who are just entering practice will have more time and incentive to learn."

One element that should be part of this collaboration is that each time a patient is referred to Dr. Li, the referring doctor should be present for the initial history, which takes up to two hours, not as a participant but as an observer. Dr. Li has told me that it is her goal, and a goal of Chinese medicine, to treat the whole person. She seeks in this first consultation to try to get a sense of not only the extent of the disease but also the underlying pathology that may be contributing to the disease's severity before she concludes whether she can help someone. This is a two-way street—the patient must also have confidence in her. Such individuation may take the direction of the first meeting down several paths. It may lead in some instances to an acupuncture treatment, as in the case of Julie, whose very real experience of repeated anaphylaxis had led to extreme anxiety. (Acupuncture, as mentioned above, is one of the few alternative treatments that has earned limited approval by NCCAM and is reimbursable by many health insurance companies.) Or the initial visit may be all talk and examination.

Enthralled though I am with Dr. Li's approach, I recognize that this kindly doctor, time-is-no-object history isn't something that only TCM practitioners do. I have watched my cousin take long histories from new patients (with their permission for me to observe), and I have seen the part it can play in gaining patient confidence as well as gaining valuable clues to patient allergies. In Dr. Groopman's book *How Doctors Think*, he recounts several cases in which patients have been studied and treated unsuccessfully for months or *years* and have achieved a breakthrough only when a new and wise doctor ignores reams of charts and tests and asks the patient to begin at the beginning. Groopman and Dr. Lisa Sanders place great stock in the importance of narrative and feeling in diagnosis.

Although healers of various scientific traditions may have many things in common, there are differences among them and strengths in each. Dr. Li says, "Western medicine is great in some areas such as surgery and infectious diseases, and TCM is great in others." The instance of EoE is a case in point of the limitations of the Western approach. Avoidance is a sensible strategy as far as it goes, and so is the use of steroids for flares, but EoE and probably all other food allergies are digestive diseases as well as immune disorders, and so the TCM approach is to treat the digestive tract as well as practicing avoidance and immune suppression. TCM practitioners look at eczema and see several possible diseases involving different parts of the body. Treating the skin with steroids while avoiding allergenic triggers only goes so far. Jackie's history (see previous chapter) reads like a kind of guide to the medical schools of the Ivy League. These doctors, like my cousin, did their best, but the patient didn't get better until she worked with Dr. Li.

Dr. Li comes to these initial meetings prepared not only to take a long history and to gain the confidence of both patient and parents, but also with a command of what amounts to an entirely new set of tools for treatment, although of course they are not new to her. This is the original holistic medicine.

To conclude, I turn again to Dr. Engler, who told me: "We have lost connection with patient stories. Patients who don't fit are marginalized. Doctors should expand their medical toolbox for patients who don't fall within guidelines. We need a mechanism for compassionate trials. Dr. Li's work is a flag in the desert. It's beautiful science."

Appendix
What It Is Like to Participate in a FAHF-2 Clinical Trial—
One Mother's Account

(Note—this account is for information about the process and its effects on a participant. The results of this trial have not yet been published.)

The FAHF-2 clinical trials are blind and anonymous from the medical side; however, there's nothing to stop participants and their families from discussing their experience, and with the instant publication opportunities afforded by the Internet, their thoughts can find a worldwide audience. One mother writing as Food Allergy Bitch (FAB) has chronicled her son's participation in a FAHF-2 trial. I reached out to her through her Twitter account, and she wrote back to me through an anonymous e-mail account.

FAB's son—I'll call him Sam—was allergic to cow's milk, soy, peanuts, and most peas and beans. FAB kept current with research through a support board she ran online, dismissing OIT trials because "we had heard from people participating how difficult it was to keep the allergen in the diet each day and how tolerances could just suddenly shift, resulting in serious reactions." When allergist Dr. Sakina Bajowala wrote favorably about FAHF-2 in her blog, The Allergist Mommy,[125] FAB decided to apply. A complete two-day examination included spirometry, a cardiac assessment, blood work, and SPT. The crux of the screening was a placebo-controlled peanut challenge—ground peanut disguised by applesauce or plain applesauce for the placebo—to find out if he was truly peanut allergic. His threshold for peanut going in was high enough that, unlike for many other peanut-allergic patients, cross-contamination was not considered a mortal threat.

FAB writes, "They were very cautious with my son because he tends to have slow-building reactions—it took a full 15 minutes on the SPT before his wheal showed up. They left a lot of time between doses to make sure everything wouldn't suddenly hit him." Despite low IgE numbers and moderate skin reactions to peanut during the screening, the young man exhibited escalating reactions as larger doses were given, and the challenge was terminated at a level of three peanuts. (A complete and vivid account of this experience is available on FAB's blog.[126])

Responding to my questions, FAB describes her son's state of mind as the trial began: "He didn't have a lot of hope about it. I think one surprising thing I've learned from all of this is that he's made his peace with the life he has to lead. He expects to be allergic to cow's milk the rest of his life, which severely limits his ability to eat out. He did the trial because he really believed he was helping science, not because he expected a miracle cure." For herself: "My fears were the obvious ones: I knew he was going to have to go through at least three reactions. The doctors assured us over and over again that there would be as little danger as possible, but of course you're always thinking about the one-in-a-million chance when you're a mom. The other fear was that my son would resent me for putting him through all of it. I do feel like I was the one pushing."

As discussed, compliance presented a series of challenges: Ten pills slightly bigger than M&Ms three times a day, ideally at least four hours apart and with meals. "He was a typical teenager and we started this trial in April, so much of the medication dosing happened over the summer. That could mean his last meal was 6:00 with the family, or at 11:00 at night depending on his work and social schedule." His high school was very strict. "We needed a letter from the trial and he had to take his lunch dose in the nurse's office each day. She was really great about it all, though, and really interested in the trial itself, as there are many other kids in the school with allergies."

Each dose was documented for the study in a log, and when he spent a week at camp, FAB tore a week of the log out and sent it, along with his pills, with him. The camp was much more relaxed about his regimen than the high school.

For six months, taking 30 pills a day, Sam kept a journal as part of the trial, but he really didn't notice any notable side effects, gastric or otherwise. After six months were up, he returned for the same round of applesauce with peanut powder. This time, he was able to eat the equivalent of nine peanuts.

Three months after Sam stopped taking the medication, he returned to see if the gains had been maintained. "They had," FAB reports. "He got to the dose just below the dose he achieved in October. He might have been able to push to one more, but there's an art to making sure these kids don't tip over into a serious reaction, and the researchers are cautious about not exceeding that magic window."

For this family, however, peanuts were not the crucial allergen. Would the protection extend to his big one—milk? Prior to the trial, Sam underwent a challenge and was able to tolerate milk in some forms: small amounts of baked milk, but not baked cheese, with some oral reactions during the challenge. All forms of milk were avoided during therapy, but afterward, food with baked milk and butter were introduced to his diet without incident.

Another big allergen for Sam was soy, which had resulted in an epinephrine injection and a trip to the ER during his freshman year in high school. "In February, we took him in for a soy challenge at his regular allergist. He passed! He has successfully added soy back into his diet at this point, although again, we're proceeding cautiously. However, he's eating Ramen noodles almost daily and has added a number of processed Chinese foods."

FAB says, "My overall assessment of participating is positive ... and wishy-washy." While she believes they have seen real benefits from the medication, she acknowledges that those benefits may not extend to all patients. "The study results are due out soon, and hopefully we'll know then whether this treatment will be appropriate for all individuals with food allergies. There are no firm answers at the end. The work that's being done is for the benefit of science and any benefit to your child is almost incidental. You don't know if it will work, or how it works. We do not have any specific instructions about how to proceed now that the trial is done. We are all waiting to see, once the results are published, if it was a success."

End notes

1. James Reston, New York Times, July 26, 1971, http://www.acupuncture.com/testimonials/restonexp.htm

2. Scott H. Sicherer, MD. Epidemiology of Food Allergy, *The Journal of Allergy and Clinical Immunology*. Volume 127, Issue 3, Pages 594–602, March 2011

3. http://www.cdc.gov/media/releases/2011/p0503_vitalsigns.html

4. http://www.worldallergy.org/publications/wao_white_book.pdf

5. http://www.ncbi.nlm.nih.gov/pmc/articles/PMC2615278/

6. Gupta et al. http://www.medpagetoday.com/MeetingCoverage/ACAAI/35940

7. Mark Jackson. *Allergy: The History of a Modern Malady*. Reaktion Books Ltd. 2006. London Page 28

8. Jonathan I. Silverberg, MD, PhD, MPH, et al. Prevalence of Allergic Disease in Foreign-Born American Children. *JAMA Pediatrics* 2013. Pages 1–7. doi:10.1001/jamapediatrics.2013.1319

9. Susan Prescott, MD. *The Allergy Epidemic*. UWA Publishing. 2011

10. Jackson, *op cit.*, p. 27

11. Jerome Groopman, MD. *How Doctors Think*. First Mariner Books. 2008. Page 122

12. http://en.wikipedia.org/wiki/Immunoglobulin_E#cite_ref-8

13. Soheila J. Maleki, PhD; Si-Yin Chung, PhD; Elaine T. Champagne, PhD; Jean-Pierre Raufman, MD. The Effects of Roasting on the Allergenic Properties of Peanut Proteins. *The Journal of Allergy and Clinical Immunology*, Volume 106, Issue 4 , Pages 763–768, October 2000

14. http://en.wikipedia.org/wiki/Protein_domain

15. B.P. Bielory; T. John; L. Bielory. Allergic Reactions to Common Allergens May Be Due to Evolutionary Immune Response to Conserved Domains (CDs) Present in Parasites and Allergens. *Journal of Allergy and Clinical Immunology*, Vol. 117, Issue 2, Supplement, Page S117, February 2006

16. Kiyoshi Hirahara, MD, PhD; Amanda Poholek, PhD; Golnaz Vahedi, PhD; Arian Laurence, PhD; Yuka Kanno, MD, PhD; Joshua D. Milner, MD; John J. O'Shea, MD. Mechanisms Underlying Helper T-cell Plasticity: Implications for Immune-Mediated Disease. *The Journal of Allergy and Clinical Immunology*, Volume 131, Issue 5, Pages 1276–1287, May 2013

17. Anne K. Ellis, MD; Michelle L. North, PhD. http://www.asthmaallergieschildren.com/2012/11/06/do-allergies-develop-in-the-womb/

18. John S. Torday, PhD; Virender K. Rehan, MD. An Epigenetic "Smoking Gun" for Reproductive Inheritance." *Expert Review of Obstetrics & Gynecology*, Volume 8, Issue 2, Pages 99–101, 2013

19. Danilo Di Bona, MD, PhD; Antonella Plaia, PhD; Maria Stefania Leto-Barone, MD; Simona La Piana, MD; Gabriele Di Lorenzo, MD. Efficacy of Subcutaneous and Sublingual Immunotherapy with Grass Allergens for Seasonal Allergic Rhinitis: A Meta-analysis–Based Comparison. *The Journal of Allergy and Clinical Immunology*, Volume 130, Issue 5, Pages 1097-1107, November 2012

20. Menno A. Kiel, MD, MSc; Esther Röder, MD, PhD; Roy Gerth van Wijk, MD, PhD; Maiwenn J. Al, PhD; Wim C.J. Hop, PhD; Maureen P.M.H. Rutten-van Mölken, PhD. Real-Life Compliance and Persistence among Users of Subcutaneous and Sublingual Allergen Immunotherapy. *The Journal of Allergy and Clinical Immunology*, Volume 132, Issue 2, Pages 353–360, August 2013; and DiBona et al., *op cit.*

21. https://web.emmes.com/study/cofar/

22. Paul M. Ehrlich. *Asthma Allergies Children: A Parent's Guide*, Page. 163 New York, Third Avenue Books 2010

23. Tse Wen Chang, PhD; Yu-Yu Shiung, BSc. Anti-IgE as a Mast Cell–Stabilizing Therapeutic Agent. *The Journal of Allergy and Clinical Immunology*, Volume 117, Issue 6 , Pages 1203–1212, June 2006

24. Volker Scheid; Dan Bensky; Andrew Ellis; Randall Barolet. *Chinese Herbal Medicine Formulas & Strategies*, 2nd edition. Eastland Press Seattle, 2009

25. Julia Ann Wisniewski, MD; Xiu-Min Li, MD, MS. Alternative and Complementary Treatment for Food Allergy. *Immunology and Allergy Clinics of North America*, Volume 32, Pages 135–150, 2012. doi:10.1016/j.iac.2011.11.001

26. Xiu-Min Li, MD; LaVerne Browne, PhD. Efficacy and Mechanisms of Action of Traditional Chinese Medicines for Treating Asthma and Allergy. *The Journal of Allergy and Clinical Immunology*, Volume 123, Issue 2, Pages 297–306, February 2009

27. http://en.wikipedia.org/wiki/Diosgenin

28. http://www.asthmaallergieschildren.com/2013/04/18/food-aller-gies-taking-the-long-view/

29. Renata J. M. Engler,, MD, FAAAAI, FACAAI; Catherine M. With, JD, LLM, LLM; Philip J. Gregory, PharmD; Jeff M. Jellin, PharmD. Complementary and Alternative Medicine for the Allergist-Immunologist: Where Do I Start? *The Journal of Allergy and Clinical Immunology*, Volume 123, Issue 2, Pages 309–316, February 2009

30. Jimmy Ko, MD; Jennifer I. Lee, MD; Anne Munoz-Furlong, BA; Xiu-Min Li, MD; Scott H. Sicherer, MD. Use of Complementary and Alternative Medicine by Food-Allergic Patients. *Annals of Allergy, Asthma & Immunology*, Pages 365-369 Volume 97, September 2006

31. T. Mainardi; Simi Kapoor; L. Bielory. Complementary and Alternative Medicine: Herbs, Phytochemicals and Vitamins and Their Immunologic Effects. *The Journal of Allergy and Clinical Immunology*, Volume 123, Issue 2, Pages 283–294, February 2009

32. Leonard Bielory. Complementary and Alternative Interventions in Asthma, Allergy, and Immunology. *Annals of Allergy and Immunology*, Volume 93, Issue 2, Supplement, Pages S45–S54, August 2004

33. Renata J. M. Engler, MD. Alternative and Complementary Medicine: A Source of Improved Therapies for Asthma? A Challenge for Redefining the Specialty? *The Journal of Allergy and Clinical Immunology*, Volume 106, Issue 4, Pages 627–629, October 2000

34. Wisniewski and Li, *op cit.*

35. Xiu-Min Li, MD. Traditional Chinese Herbal Remedies for Asthma and Food Allergy. *Journal of Allergy and Clinical Immunology* volume 120, number 1 2007 pp. 25-31

36. J. O. Lee; J. Y. Lee; Y. H. Ahn; Y. Han; K. Ahn; S. I. Lee. Ara h2 Is Not a Major Peanut Allergen in Korea. *The Journal of Allergy and Clinical Immunology*, Volume 125, Issue 2, Supplement 1, Page AB225, February 2010

37. Xiu-Min Li; Chih-Kang Huang; Brian H. Schofield; A. Wesley Burks; Gary A. Bannon; Kawn-Hyoung Kim; Shau-Ku Huang; Hugh A. Sampson. Strain-Dependent Induction of Allergic Sensitization Caused by Peanut Allergen DNA Immunization in Mice *Journal of Immunology*, Volume 162, Pages3045–3052, 1999

38. http://www.ehow.com/facts_5576289_roundworms-life-cycle-humans.html

39. S. Nagaraji; R. Raghavan; R. Macaden; A.V. Kurpad. Intestinal Parasitic Infection and Total Serum IgE in Asymtomatic Adult Males in an Urban Slum and Efficacy of Antiparasitic Therapy. *Indian Journal of Medical Microbology*, Volume 22, Issue 1, Pages 54–56, 2004

40. Michael Gurish et al. *The Journal of Immunology*, Volume 172, Issue 2, Pages 1139–1145, January 15, 2004, http://www.jimmunol.org/content/172/2/1139.full

41. Xiu-Min Li. Traditional Chinese Herbal Remedies for Asthma and Food Allergy. *Journal of Allergy and Clinical Immunology*, Volume 120, Number 1 Pages 25-31, p. 29

42. Richard S. H. Pumphrey; Ian S. D. Roberts. Postmortem Findings after Fatal Anaphylactic Reactions. *Journal of Clinical Pathology*, Volume 53, Pages :273–276, 2000

43. Outcomes of the European Commission Workshop "Are Mice Relevant Models for Human Disease?" held in London, UK, on 21 May 2010, http://ec.europa.eu/research/health/pdf/summary-report-25082010_en.pdf

44. Engler, With, Gregory, Jellin, op cit. p. 312

45. Xiu-Min Li, MD; Denise Serebrisky, MD; Soo-Young Lee, MD; Chih-Kang Huang, MS; Ludmilla Bardina, MS; Brian H. Schofield, JD; J. Steven Stanley, PhD; A. Wesley Burks, MD; Gary A. Bannon, PhD; Hugh A. Sampson, MD. A Murine Model of Peanut Anaphylaxis: T- and B-cell Responses to a Major Peanut Allergen Mimic

Human Responses *Journal of Allergy and Clinical Immunology*, Volume 106, Issue 1, Part 1 pages 150-158

46. http://jaxmice.jax.org/strain/000659.html

47. http://en.wikipedia.org/wiki/Cholera

48. Y. Fang; L. Larsson; J. Mattsson; N. Lycke; Z. Xiang. Mast Cells Contribute to the Mucosal Adjuvant Effect of CTA1-DD after IgG-complex Formation. *Journal of Immunology*, Volume 185, Issue 5, Pages 2935–2941, September 2010. doi: 10.4049/jimmunol.1000589. Epub 2010 Jul 30.

49. Joaquín Sánchez; Jan Holmgren. Cholera Toxin: A Friend & Foe. *Indian Journal of Medical Research* Volume 133, Issue 2, Pages 153–163, February 2011

50. John Chen; Tina Chen. Chapter 7, *Chinese Medical Herbology and Pharmacology*. Art of Medicine Press. 2004. City of Industry, Ca. http://www.aompress.com/book_herbology/pdfs/FuZi.pdf

51. Xiu-Min Li, MD Teng-Fei Zhang, PhD Chih-Kang Huang, M.S.Kamal Srivastava, BSªAriel A. Teper, MD Libang Zhang, MD Brian H. Schofield, JD Hugh A. Sampson, MD *The Journal of Allergy and Clinical Immunology Food Allergy Herbal Formula-1 (FAHF-1) blocks peanut-induced anaphylaxis in a murinemodel* Volume 108, Issue 4, Pages 639-646, October 2001

52. http://en.wikipedia.org/wiki/Ephedra

53. http://en.wikipedia.org/wiki/Datura_stramonium

54. http://www.fda.gov/OHRMS/DOCKETS/98fr/001392gd.pdf

55. http://www.bing.com/Dictionary/search?q=define+aconitine& qpvt=acontine&FORM=DTPDIA

56. http://www.fda.gov/Food/DietarySupplements/Alerts/ucm096388.htm

57. Kamal D. Srivastava, MPhil, Jacob D. Kattan, BS, Zhong Mei Zou, PhD, Jing Hua Li, MD, Libang Zhang, MD,b Sylvan Wallenstein, PhD, Joseph Goldfarb, PhD, Hugh A. Sampson, MD, and Xiu-Min Li, MD The Chinese herbal medicine formula FAHF-2 completely blocks anaphylactic reactions in a murine model of peanut allergy *J Allergy Clin Immunol January* 2005 171-178

58. http://en.wikipedia.org/wiki/Normal_human_body_temperature

59. [i] C. Qu; K. Srivastava; J. Ko; T. F. Zhang; H. A. Sampson; X-M. Li.

Induction of tolerance after establishment of peanut allergy by the food allergy herbal formula-2 is associated with up-regulation of interferon-g *Clinical and Experimental Allergy*, Volume 37, Pages 846–855

60. Following the final challenge, splenocytes and mesenteric lymph node (MLN) cells derived from each group were isolated by gently grinding spleens or MLNs using a syringe plunger and were strained through nylon (BD Biosciences, Bedford, MA, USA). After lysis—deconstruction—of red blood cells, splenocytes or MLN cells were re-suspended in RPMI 1640 "series of media using a bicarbonate buffering system and alterations in the amounts of amino acids and vitamins"supplemented with 10% FBS (fetal bovine serum). Cells were cultured, and after 72 hours, liquids also known as supernatants were separated from the various cytokines, including IL-4, IL-5, IL-13, IL-10, TGF-b, and IFN-γ. These were measured using the ELISA test determined by ELISA in triplicate according to the manufacturer's instructions using companies in three different states for particular components (R&D Systems, Minneapolis, MN, USA, for IL-13; Promega, Madison, WI, USA, for TGF-b; and BD Pharmingen, San Diego, CA, USA, for all others).

61. Victor Turcanu; Soheila J. Maleki; Gideon Lack. Characterization of Lymphocyte Responses to Peanuts in Normal Children, Peanut-Allergic Children, and Allergic Children Who Acquired Tolerance to Peanuts. *Journal of Clinical Investigation*, Volume 111, Issue 7, Pages 1065–1072, April 1, 2003

62. Ehrlich, et al., *op cit.*, p. 114

63. J. Bellanti et al. *Immunology IV: Clinical Applications in Health and Disease.* Care Press Bethesda, MD. 2012

64. Li; Brown, *op cit.p. 301*

65. Jacob D. Kattan; Kamal D. Srivastava; Zhong Mei Zou; Joseph Goldfarb; Hugh A. Sampson; Xiu-Min Li. Pharmacological and Immunological Effects of Individual Herbs in the Food Allergy Herbal Formula-2 (FAHF-2) on Peanut Allergy. *Phytotherapy Research*, Volume 22, Issue 5, May 2008, Pages: 651–659 p. 658

66. Changda Liu; Nan Yang; Ying Song; Lixin Wang; Jiachen Zi; Bingji Ma; David Dunkin; Keith Benkov; Clare Ceballos; Paula Busse; Jody Tversky; Hugh Sampson; Joseph Goldfarb; Jixun Zhan; Xiu-Min Li.. manuscript in preparation

67. http://allergicliving.com/index.php/2013/03/13/milk-oral-immunotherapy-not-lasting/

68. Kamal D. Srivastava, MPhil, Jacob D. Kattan, BS, Zhong Mei Zou, PhD, Jing Hua Li, MD, Libang Zhang, MD,b Sylvan Wallenstein, PhD, Joseph Goldfarb, PhD, Hugh A. Sampson, MD, and Xiu-Min Li, MD The Chinese herbal medicine formula FAHF-2 completely blocks anaphylactic reactions in a murine model of peanut allergy *J Allergy Clin Immunol January* 2005 171-178 . 171

69. Prednisone and Other Corticosteroids. http://www.mayo-clinic.com/health/steroids/HQ01431

70. http://en.wikipedia.org/wiki/TGF_beta

71. Kamal D. Srivastava, MPhil; Chunfeng Qu, MD, PhD; Tengfei Zhang, PhD; Joseph Goldfarb, PhD; Hugh A. Sampson, MD; Xiu-Min Li, MD. Food Allergy Herbal Formula-2 Silences Peanut-Induced Anaphylaxis for a Prolonged Posttreatment Period via IFN-g–Producing CD8+ T Cells. *Journal of Allergy and Clinical Immunology*, Volume 123, Issue 2, February 2009

72. Kiyoshi Hirahara, MD, PhD; Amanda Poholek, PhD; Golnaz Vahedi, PhD; Arian Laurence, PhD, MRCP; Yuka Kanno, MD, PhD; Joshua D. Milner, MD; John J. O'Shea, MD. Mechanisms Underlying Helper T-cell Plasticity: Implications for Immune-Mediated Disease. *The Journal of Allergy and Clinical Immunology*, Volume 131, Issue 5, Pages 1276–1287, May 2013

73. Julie Wang; Sangita P. Patil; Nan Yang; Jimmy Ko; Joohee Lee; Sally Noone; Hugh A. Sampson; Xiu-Min Li. Safety, Tolerability, and Immunologic Effects of a Food Allergy Herbal Formula in Food Allergic Individuals: A Randomized, Double-Blinded, Placebo-Controlled, Dose Escalation, Phase 1 Study. *Annals of Allergy, Asthma & Immunology*, Volume 105, Issue 1, Pages 75–84, July 2010

74. Sangita P. Patil, PhD; Julie Wang, MD; Ying Song, MD; Sally Noone, RN; Nan Yang, PhD; Sylvan Wallenstein, PhD; Hugh A. Sampson, MD; Xiu-Min Li, MD. Clinical Safety of Food Allergy Herbal Formula-2 (FAHF-2) and Inhibitory Effect on Basophils from Patients with Food Allergy: Extended Phase I Study. *Journal of Allergy and Clinical Immunology*, Volume 128, Issue 6, Pages 1259–1265 Dec. 2011

75. S. M. Jones; L. Pons; J. L. Roberts; A. M. Scurlock; T. T. Perry; M. Kulis, et al. Clinical Efficacy and Immune Regulation with Peanut

Oral Immunotherapy. *Journal of Allergy & Clinical Immunology*, Volume 124, Pages 292–300, 2009

76. http://www.sciencedaily.com/releases/2012/06/120625125952.htm?utm_source=feedburner&utm_medium=email&utm_campaign=Feed%3A+sciencedaily%2Fhealth_medicine%2Fallergy+%28Science Daily%3A+Health+%26+Medicine+News+—+Allergy%29

77. http://allergicliving.com/index.php/2012/04/27/time-to-end-food-allergy-tragedies/?page=2

78. K. Srivastava; N. Yang; Y. Chen; I. Lopez-Exposito; Y. Song; J. Goldfarb; J. Zhan; H. Sampson; and X-M. Li. Efficacy, Safety and Immunological Actions of Butanol-Extracted Food Allergy Herbal Formula-2 on Peanut Anaphylaxis. *Clinical & Experimental Allergy*, Volume 41, Issue 4, April 2011, Pages: 582–591

79. 1. Definitely related: An AE that follows a temporal sequence from administration of the test product and/or procedure; follows a known response pattern to the test article and/or procedure; and, when appropriate to the protocol, is confirmed by improvement after stopping the test product and cannot be reasonably explained by known characteristics of the subject's clinical state or by other therapies.

2. Probably related: An AE that follows a reasonable temporal sequence from administration of the test product and/or procedure; follows a known response pattern to the test product and/or procedure; and cannot be reasonably explained by the known characteristics of the participant's clinical state or other therapies.

3. Possibly related: An AE that follows a reasonable temporal sequence from administration of the test product and/or procedure and follows a known response pattern to the test product and/or procedure, but could have been produced by the participant's clinical state or by other therapies.

Not associated: An AE for which sufficient information exists to indicate that the etiology is not related to the test product and/or therapy.

Unrelated: An AE that does not follow a reasonable temporal sequence after administration of the test product and/or procedure and most likely is explained by the participant's clinical disease state or by other therapies. (IND 77468 Phase 1 for B-FAHF-2)

80. Guidelines for the Diagnosis and Management of Food Allergy in the United States: Report of the NIAID-Sponsored Expert Panel. *The Journal of Allergy and Clinical Immunology*, Volume 126, Issue 6, Pages S1S58, December 2010

81. J. L. Brozek; L. Terracciano; J. Hsu; J. Kreis; E. Compalati; N. Santesso; et al. Oral Immunotherapy for IgE-Mediated Cow's Milk Allergy: A Systematic Review and Meta-Analysis. *Clinical & Experimental Allergy*, Volume 42, Issue 3, Pages 363–374, 2012. See more at http://www.asthmaallergieschildren.com/2012/05/11/oral-immunotherapy-for-food-allergy-not-ready-for-prime-time/#sthash.CeusCFfJ.dpuf

82. Lee et al., *op cit.*

83. S. M. Jones; L. Pons; J. L. Roberts; A. M. Scurlock; T. T. Perry; M. Kulis M; et al. Clinical Efficacy and Immune Regulation with Peanut Oral Immunotherapy. *Journal of Allergy and Clinical Immunology*, Volume 124, Issue 2, Pages 292–300, 2009

84. http://www.asthmaallergieschildren.com/2013/04/20/history-is-made-at-lunch/

85. IND 77468 Phase 1 for B-FAHF-2

86. Chris Faulk. Lamarck, Lysenko, and Modern Day Epigenetics. http://www.mindthesciencegap.org/2013/06/21/lamarck-lysenko-and-modern-day-epigenetics/

87. Kari Nadeau, MD, PhD; Cameron McDonald-Hyman, BA; Elizabeth M. Noth, PhD; Boriana Pratt, MA; S. Katharine Hammond, PhD; John Balmes, MD; Ira Tager, MD, MPH. Ambient Air Pollution Impairs Regulatory T-cell Function in Asthma. *Journal of Allergy and Clinical Immunology*, Volume 126, Issue 4, Pages 845–852, October 2010

88. John S. Torday, PhD; Virender K. Rehan, MD. Review of Obstetrics & Gynecology March 2013. *Science Daily*, March 4, 2013

89. Faulk, *op cit.*

90. Iván López-Expósito, PhD; Ying Song, MD; Kirsi M. Järvinen, MD, PhD; Kamal Srivastava, MPhil; Xiu-Min Li, MD. Maternal Peanut Exposure During Pregnancy and Lactation Reduces Peanut Allergy Risk in Offspring. *Journal of Allergy and Clinical Immunology*, Volume 124, Issue 5, Pages 1039–1049, November 2009

91. I. Lopez-Exposito; N. Birmingham; A. Castillo; X-M. Li. ASHMI (Anti-Asthma Herbal Medicine Intervention) Prevents Maternal Transmission of Early Onset of Allergic Airway Inflammation and Mucus Cell Development in Offspring (abstract). *Journal of Allergy & Clinical Immunology*, Volume 125, Issue 2, Page S120, 2010

92. Ming-Chun Wen, MD; et al. Efficacy and Tolerability of Antiasthma Herbal Medicine Intervention in Adult Patients with Moderate-Severe Allergic Asthma. *Journal of Allergy & Clinical Immunology*, Volume 116, Pages 517–524, September 2005

93. X. Li; K. Srivastava; J. Chen. ASHMI, But Not Corticosteroid Treatment Restores Maternal Allergen Long-term Tolerance and Prevents Offspring Asthma Risk via Epigenetic Modulation Control/Tracking Number: 12-LB-5741-AAAA(Abstract for proposed publication)

94. Olga Luengo, MD, PhD; Ying Song, MD; Kamal Srivastava, PhD; Xiu-Min Li, MD. The Potential of Maternal Dietary Modification for Prevention of Food Allergy [in press as of August 3, 2013]

95. Ying Song, MD; Ching-feng Huang; ChangDa Liu; Paul Faybusovich; Jia Chen, PhD; Xiu-Min Li, MD. Maternal Transmission of Peanut Allergy Susceptibility Is Associated with IL-4 Promoter Demethylation in Offspring. *Journal of Allergy & Clinical Immunology*, Volume 131, Issue 2, Supplement, Page AB218, February 2013

96. Antonella D'Ambrosio et al. Cholera toxin B subunit promotes the induction of regulatory T cells by preventing human dendritic cell maturation *Journal of Leukocyte Biology*, Volume 84, Issue 3, Pages 661–668, 2008.

97. Dr. Kari Nadeau. Turning the Tables on an Evolutionary Mistake—Stanford Researchers Go for the Cure. http://www.asthmaallergies-children.com/2012/09/21/turning-the-tables-on-an-%E2%80%9C evolutionary-mistake%E2%80%9D-%E2%80%93-stanford-researchers-go-for-the-cure/

98. http://en.wikipedia.org/wiki/Interleukin_10

99. Susan L. Prescott. Early-Life Environmental Determinants of Allergic Diseases and the Wider Pandemic of Inflammatory Noncommunicable Diseases. *Journal of Allergy & Clinical Immunology*, Volume 131, Issue 1, Pages 23–30, January 2013 p.23

100. http://ibdcrohns.about.com/cs/ibdfaqs/a/ibd101.htm

101. http://en.wikipedia.org/wiki/Crohn%27s_disease

102. J. Bellanti et al., *op cit.*

103. http://icahn.mssm.edu/research/programs/jaffe-food-allergy-institute/clinical-trials

104. http://en.wikipedia.org/wiki/Organ_transplantation

105. J. Reid-Adam; N. Yang; Y. Song; P. Cravedi; X-M. Li; P. Heeger. Immunosuppressive Effects of the Traditional Chinese Herb Qu Mai on Human Alloreactive T Cells. *American Journal of Transplantation.* Volume 13, Issue 5, pages 1159–1167, May 2013

106. Ibid p. 1159.

107. Trends in Asthma Morbidity and Mortality, American Lung Association, Epidemiology and Statistics Unit, Research and Health Education Division, September 2012

108. Wen et al., *op cit.*

109. Min-Li Hong; Ying Song; Xiu-Min Li. *Chinese Journal of Integrative Medicine*, Volume 17, Issue 7, Pages 483–491, July 2011 p. 484

110. Ibid. p. 485

111. http://www.newyorker.com/reporting/2012/04/23/120423 fa_fact_groopman#ixzz2NcyoxyDC

112. Ron Rosenbaum. "Tales from the Cancer Cure Underground." *The Secret Parts of Fortune.* Random House, New York, 2000

113. Daniel Engber Is the Cure for Cancer Inside You? *New York Times*, December 21, 2012 http://www.nytimes.com/2012/12/23/ magazine/is-the-cure-for-cancer-inside-you.html

114. Andrew Pollack Drug Helps Defense System Fight Cancer *New York Times*, June 1, 2012 http://www.nytimes.com/2012/06/02/business/drug-helps-immune-system-fight-cancer.html?_r=0

115. Denise Grady In Girl's Last Hope, Altered Immune Cells Beat Leukemia *New York Times*, December 9, 2012

116. Martin J. Walsh. Inhibition of Tumor Cell Growth by Herbal Preparation MSSM-03_(unpublished)

117. Mario Noti; Elia D. Tait Wojno; Brian S. Kim; Mark C. Siracusa; Paul R. Giacomin; Meera G. Nair; Alain J. Benitez; Kathryn R.

Ruymann; Amanda B. Muir; David A. Hill; Kudakwashe R. Chik-wava; Amin E. Moghaddam; Quentin J. Sattentau; Aneesh Alex; Chao Zhou; Jennifer H. Yearley; Paul Menard-Katcher; Masato Kubo; Kazushige Obata-Ninomiya; Hajime Karasuyama; Michael R. Comeau; Terri Brown-Whitehorn; Rene de Waal Malefyt; Patrick M. Sleiman; Hakon Hakonarson; Antonella Cianferoni; Gary W. Falk, Mei-Lun Wang; Jonathan M. Spergel; David Artis. Thymic Stromal Lymphopoietin–Elicited Basophil Responses Promote Eosinophilic Esophagitis. *Nature Medicine*, 2013 abstract— *http://www.nature.com/nm/journal/v19/n8/full/nm.3281.html.*

118. Lisa Sanders, MD. *Every Patient Tells a Story.* Broadway Books, New York, 2009

119. Groopman, *op cit. p. 219*

120. Engler et al., *op cit.*

121. Paul M. O'Byrne, MB. Asthma in the Real World. *Journal of Allergy & Clinical Immunology*, Volume 132, Issue 1, Pages 70–71, July 2013

122. Guidelines for the Diagnosis and Management of Food Allergy in the United States: Report of the NIAID-Sponsored Expert Panel. *Journal of Allergy & Clinical Immunology*, Volume 126, Issue 6, Supplement, December 2010. Section 3.4.3

123. Philip L. Lieberman; Mchael S. Blaiss. Current Medicine, Philadelphia, 2002

124. Matthew Greenhawt, MD, MBA, MSc; Seema S. Aceves, MD, PhD; Jonathan M. Spergel, MD, PhD; Marc E. Rothenberg, MD, PhD. The Management of Eosinophilic Esophagitis. *Journal of Allergy and Clinical Immunology: In Practice*, Volume 1, Issue 4, Pages 332–340, July 2013

125. http://allergistmommy.blogspot.com/2010/09/chinese-herbal-for-mula-to-protect.html

126. http://foodallergybitch.blogspot.com/2012/04/btdt-got-fahf-2-food-allergy-clinical.html